THE BETTER PERIOD FOOD SOLUTION

Eat Your Way to a Lifetime of Healthier Cycles

TRACY LOCKWOOD BECKERMAN
MS, RD, CDN

BANISH BLOAT AND BREAKOUTS, BALANCE HORMONES, AND REDUCE PAINFUL CRAMPS

ULYSSES PRESS

Published in the United States by:
ULYSSES PRESS
P.O. Box 3440
Berkeley, CA 94703
www.ulyssespress.com

ISBN: 978-1-61243-939-6
Library of Congress Control Number: 2019942124

Printed in Canada by Marquis Book Printing
10 9 8 7 6 5 4 3 2 1

Acquisitions editor: Bridget Thoreson
Managing editor: Claire Chun
Project editor: Renee Rutledge
Proofreader: Kate St. Clair
Indexer: Sayre Van Young
Front cover design: Malea Clark-Nicholson
Cover photos: © CarinhaScobeleva/shutterstock.com
Interior design and layout: what!design @ whatweb.com
Interior art: page 11 © Marochkina Anastasiia/shutterstock.com; page 59 © Elena
     Schweitzer/shutterstock.com; page 69 © Ekaterina Markelova/shutterstock.com;
     page 278 © Diana Arzoomanian

NOTE TO READERS: This book has been written and published strictly for informational and educational purposes only. It is not intended to serve as medical advice or to be any form of medical treatment. You should always consult your physician before altering or changing any aspect of your medical treatment and/or undertaking a diet regimen, including the guidelines as described in this book. Do not stop or change any prescription medications without the guidance and advice of your physician. Any use of the information in this book is made on the reader's good judgment after consulting with his or her physician and is the reader's sole responsibility. This book is not intended to diagnose or treat any medical condition and is not a substitute for a physician. This book is independently authored and published and no sponsorship or endorsement of this book by, and no affiliation with, any trademarked brands or other products mentioned within is claimed or suggested. All trademarks that appear in ingredient lists and elsewhere in this book belong to their respective owners and are used here for informational purposes only. The author and publisher encourage readers to patronize the quality brands mentioned in this book.

To all the ladies (myself included) who have had to hide tampons or pads up their sleeve on their way to the bathroom. This one's for us.

CONTENTS

INTRODUCTION

Jeans that won't zip, stubborn cheek pimples, relentless chocolate cravings, uncontrolled tears after watching tiny puppies play. Does any of this sound familiar to you? If your period had a voice, she would say, "Sweetie, it's not you, it's me." You better believe that your period and reproductive health have more control over you than you think, for better or for worse.

Because no one dares to voice the truth about their period (we've been stuck in this period suppression for eons), it's been nearly impossible to become informed and truly understand what the heck is going on down there...until NOW! This book is going to help tackle the menstruation taboo, aid in the menstrual revolution, and teach you how to nutritionally support yourself toward a better period. Period.

I want this book to empower you, squash menstrual shame, and make you feel like an absolute boss when it comes to your period. It will help you break free from the shackles society has placed on periods and menstrual health. Understanding what foods and nutrients your body needs to amplify your cycle will ignite you to support your cravings, mood swings, and hormonal fluctuations, and, finally, take control of your period—not the other way around.

A bit about me. A big reason why I even got into the field of nutrition was because I wanted to know exactly how food affects the body. No one really talks about why food makes them feel a certain way, and that didn't seem right to me. Why did some foods make me feel happy while others down in the dumps? Why did some foods make me feel tired or more energized? And why was I craving certain foods more (ahem, chocolate) right before my period? In order to find the answers I was looking for, I became a registered dietitian and pursued a master's degree in clinical nutrition from New York University.

If you don't know what a registered dietitian is, we are basically doctors of food. We dissect every metabolic system, every organ, and every medical ailment and learn how food and nutrition can prevent disease and even heal or treat a medical condition. It may sound strange but when we see food, we see medicine.

Registered dietitians are also scientists. We dissect evidence, data, and stats to compile sound, ethical, unbiased, and well-researched answers. We are required to work in hospitals and have to get matched to a dietetic internship program to complete a residency program (similar to what doctors have to go through). We also have to pass a national dietetics exam before we can legally practice as a registered dietitian. My point is, registered dietitians know what we are talking about.

I decided to specialize in women's health because I wanted to teach women how to nutritionally support their periods, enhance their fertility, and improve their reproductive health. My clients often ask me, "Is it even possible to eat your way toward a healthier menstrual cycle?" As I immediately smile, I can't help but exclaim, "Yes, it is possible!" Good nutrition can keep your reproductive system going like a well-oiled machine, powered by real foods.

Besides being professionally qualified, I personally understand how impactful nutrition (and self-care) is for a healthy menstrual cycle. After I stopped taking the pill, it took me a long time to restore my natural menstrual cycle. Like an old iPhone that hasn't been powered in years, I had to adjust my lifestyle, eating patterns, and, ultimately, my perspective of health to bring my period back to life.

I was in need of real, science-based nutrition facts while I was going through my own journey; something relatable, digestible (pun intended!), and evidenced based, and I did not have anywhere trustworthy to lean on. This book will ultimately fill that gap as it tackles the topic of nutrition for periods, so think of it as my gift to you. I hope this book will empower you to lean in toward FOOD as medicine to help you "surf the crimson wave," as Cher Horowitz from *Clueless* puts it, and feel even more like a fearless female (though you already are!).

This book will introduce you to "food cycling," a novel concept I created that's been extremely beneficial for women to help understand their bodies and their menstrual cycles better. Food cycling teaches the importance of eating particular nutrients during each phase of the cycle to promote hormonal balance, enhance well-being, manage mood, reduce premenstrual syndrome (PMS), and boost energy. Certain phases during your cycle mess with your appetite, mood for specific foods, sexual desire, and even your personality. This book gives you guidelines on how to work within those parameters rather than trying to escape them. No matter if you are 13 or 45, studies upon studies have shown that food cravings and even our appetite is influenced through feisty hormones that ebb and flow during our cycle. Regardless of age, we should all learn how and why hormones have the ability to magically transport us from our couch to our kitchen. *Speaking on behalf of a friend! :)*

I'll also teach you which nutrients manage and heal symptoms in reproductive and hormonal conditions such as polycystic ovarian syndrome (PCOS), endometriosis, amenorrhea, and PMS, all backed by evidence-based research. This book also lays the ropes of fertility-focused nutrition to help those who want to be proactive in supporting their bodies toward an optimal environment for future pregnancies.

Society has placed a taboo surrounding periods and menstrual health, as if we should be ashamed of this natural and miraculous process that's ultimately kept the human species alive. We have to be more open about the topic of good period health and break the stigma, one voice at a time. No longer should we be embarrassed to talk about our periods, our cramps, our moodiness, our pain, or our struggles to get our cycles back or become pregnant. For crying out loud, the documentary *Period. End of Sentence* won an Oscar this year! Ladies, let's end this nonsense and let's talk about it, learn about it, and do something about it. Let's be part of the change and make menstruation mainstream. Us gals have to stick together, right?

PERIOD 101

Before we dive into the best foods to eat to support a healthier period, let's learn more about the endocrine (the collection of glands that produce hormones) and reproductive systems, and how they play in the same sandbox as the menstrual cycle.

Our body is more connected than you may think. There are conversations going on 24/7 between our nervous system, digestive system, and endocrine system through little sound bites known as neurotransmitters. These chemical messengers dictate basically everything, such as behavior, mood, sleep, and so much more. In addition to neurotransmitters, our body is controlled through something we are all very familiar with: hormones!

HORMONAL HELPERS

The menstrual cycle is truly a physiological miracle made possible through the dedication of hormones. It's a tightly coordinated cycle that relies on precise hormonal symbiosis and timing. Think of your hormones as a cheerleading squad—all cheerleaders need to be in sync and work together to successfully perform those jaw-dropping stunts!

Hormones communicate through the blood and nervous system and basically have VIP access to all the cells in the body. These hardworking hormones tightly regulate the endocrine system to maintain homeostasis, or natural balance, in the body. Their effects can take as little as seconds or as long as days to be felt. Pretty cool stuff!

Hormones are carried through the blood to all parts of the body to initiate a menstrual cycle. Hormonal signals fire off in the hypothalamus, a pea-sized controller in the brain that sits pretty at the top of the menstrual hierarchy. Think of the hypothalamus as Beyoncé, the ultimate decision-maker and leader. Beyoncé interprets what's going on in the body and then says yah or nah to specific hormone production in the bod. Her answer has a domino effect on *a lot* of menstrual cycle decisions thereafter. Imagine Beyoncé instructing her personal assistant to coordinate with her glam squad (e.g., stylist, hair and makeup team) to create the best looks for an upcoming music video. Her posse needs to work together to come up with knockout costumes and styles and then depend on the final approval from upper management, aka Queen Bey, before moving forward. So yes, a lot of peeps are involved!

Trudging forth with our menstrual cycle class...hormones are carried to the pituitary gland, basically Beyoncé's right-hand man (or should I say woman!). Hormones are then secreted at various sites thereafter: gonadotropin-releasing hormone (GnRH) is secreted by the hypothalamus; follicle-stimulating hormone (FSH) and luteinizing hormone (LH) are secreted by the pituitary gland; and estrogen and progesterone are secreted by the ovaries.

FSH and LH signal ovulation (when the ovaries release an egg). Afterward, a surge in estrogen and progesterone promotes thick uterine tissue to grow in the uterus to potentially support a pregnancy. If pregnancy does not occur, estrogen and progesterone plummet and voilà! your period arrives as your uterine lining sheds. This entire process takes place every month (unless you become pregnant or enter menopause).

Many more hormones are involved in the picture, such as testosterone, androgen, thyroid-stimulating hormone (TSH), parathyroid hormone (PTH), adrenocorticotropic hormone (ACTH), prolactin, glucagon, insulin, cortisol, adrenaline, calcitonin, and human growth hormone (see the Hormonal Breakdown chart on page 8 for more information). These, and many others, work together to facilitate a menstrual cycle by acting on glands, such as the adrenal gland, thyroid gland, parathyroid gland, and of course, the ovaries!

There is a lot of responsibility riding on the ovaries every month. The ovaries need to coordinate with the rest of the endocrine squad (hormones, glands, and organs) and be ready each month to prep the body for the undertaking of a potential pregnancy. As you can imagine, this process requires precise hormonal coordination during every single menstrual cycle, even if pregnancy does not occur.

Hormonal Breakdown

HORMONE	FUNCTION	SECRETION GLAND
Gonadotropin-releasing hormone (GnRH)	Releases follicle-stimulating hormone (FSH) and luteinizing hormone (LH), which control the menstrual cycle and ovulation.	Hypothalamus
Adrenocorticotropic hormone (ACTH)	Triggers the release of cortisol and androgen hormones.	Pituitary gland
Follicle-stimulating hormone (FSH)	Stimulates the growth of follicles in the ovaries before the release of an egg from one follicle during ovulation.	Pituitary gland
Human growth hormone (HGH)	Promotes growth in children and helps adults properly utilize fat and protein for energy.	Pituitary gland
Luteinizing hormone (LH)	Involved in puberty, ovulation, and pregnancy. An "LH surge" triggers ovulation during the cycle.	Pituitary gland
Prolactin	Promotes milk production after childbirth.	Pituitary gland
Calcitonin	Regulates calcium levels, particularly if calcium is building up in the body.	Thyroid
Thyroid-stimulating hormone (TSH)	Impacts metabolism. Altered levels of TSH may lead to hyperthyroidism (abnormally fast metabolism) or hypothyroidism (abnormally slow metabolism).	Thyroid
Parathyroid hormone (PTH)	Regulates the amount of calcium and phosphorous in the body, particularly if calcium levels are low.	Parathyroid gland
Insulin	Moves the sugar we consume as food into our body's cells for use as energy.	Pancreas
Glucagon	Creates energy from compounds within the body when a food source is not available.	Pancreas

Hormonal Breakdown

HORMONE	FUNCTION	SECRETION GLAND
Adrenaline	Known as the "fight-or-flight hormone"; allows the body to effectively use energy in stressful or even life-threatening situations.	Adrenal gland
Cortisol	Known as the "stress hormone"; released in response to stress and maintains blood sugar levels, regulates metabolism, and reduces inflammation.	Adrenal gland
Androgen	A class of hormones that promotes the development of the reproductive system and functioning, facilitates puberty, regulates emotional well-being and sexual drive, and plays a role in estrogen production.	Ovaries
Estrogen	Responsible for the development and regulation of the reproductive system and menstrual cycle. There are three forms of estrogen: estradiol, estrone, and estriol, and estradiol is the most biologically active and potent form of estrogen in women.	Ovaries and adipose tissue
Progesterone	Helps to thicken the lining of the uterus (endometrium) every month to support a potential pregnancy after ovulation.	Ovaries, adrenal gland, and placenta (if pregnant)
Testosterone	Regulates sex drive, reproductive tissue, body composition, and bone growth. Yes, women have testosterone too!	Ovaries

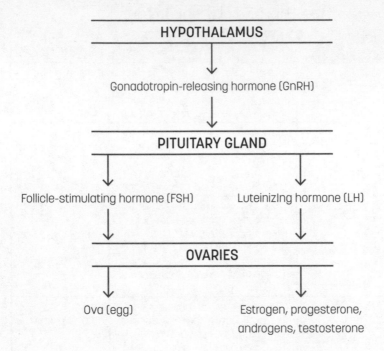

Hormones are extremely sensitive, but don't worry, that's a good thing! Hormones are influenced by a plethora of factors including the foods we eat, stress levels, lack of sleep, age, medication, and environmental conditions, such as light and temperature. The hypothalamus responds to these factors and then tells the body to either make more or less of that hormone. For example, the hypothalamus is impacted tremendously by anxiety. Anxiety has the power to inhibit the release of the hormone oxytocin, which is known as the "love hormone." So, when you are feeling anxious it's no wonder you aren't feeling so lovey dovey!

THE MENSTRUAL CYCLE DEETS

The goal of the menstrual cycle is to release a single, mature ova (egg) from a huge pool of eggs. This is how the cycle works:

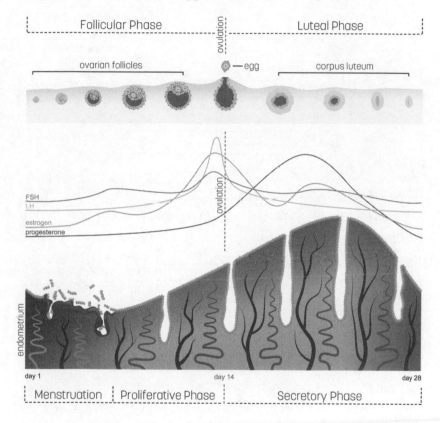

The Menstrual Cycle in Action

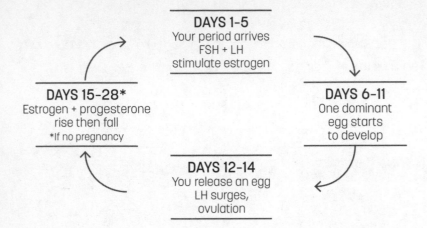

DAYS 1-5
Your period arrives
FSH + LH
stimulate estrogen

DAYS 15-28*
Estrogen + progesterone
rise then fall
*If no pregnancy

DAYS 6-11
One dominant
egg starts
to develop

DAYS 12-14
You release an egg
LH surges,
ovulation

Believe it or not, each and every month the body is prepared to support a pregnancy. When pregnancy doesn't occur, your period comes. A menstrual cycle can be anywhere from 21 days to 35 days. Your cycle is measured from the first day of your last period to the first day of your next period. For example, day 1 of your cycle is the first day of bleeding.

The menstrual cycle is not black and white. Meaning, some women could have a shorter or longer cycle, could menstruate for longer than five days, could ovulate anywhere from days 10 to 18, or could have PMS the day after they ovulate or the day before their period. I'm basing the following breakdown around a 28-day cycle as a general average cycle length, but from woman to woman, there is a lot of variation. The timing below is an approximation because the menstrual cycle is not an exact science. Remember that everyone's bodies are beautiful and uniquely different, just be aware of your own!

Based on an average 28-day cycle, to further break it down:

1. Menstrual Phase (days 1-5), you bleed

2. Follicular Phase (days 6-11), getting ready to release an egg

3. Ovulatory Phase (days 12-14), releasing of the egg

4. Luteal Phase (days 15-28), getting ready to bleed...again. FYI, PMS can start any time after ovulation until menses onset.

DISCLAIMER: To help you separate the phases of your cycle with hopes of learning what distinct nutrients your body needs, I've decided to chop up the phases this way. Although, you've probably learned that the follicular phase is considered the first half of your cycle, starts on the first day of your cycle, refers to all the days prior to ovulation, and could last more than 2 weeks depending on when you ovulate. Please see Follicular Phase on page 33 for more information.

NEW PHASE, WHO THIS?

The reproductive system is anything but basic. Each phase is roped together with intricate ups and downs that are associated with physical, emotional, cognitive, mood, sleep, and hormonal changes. You know on *The Bachelor* when the contestants describe the journey as an emotional roller coaster? Well, like the show, each phase of the cycle is a different and wild adventure. My advice? Hold on!

Jokes aside, each phase of the cycle is associated with different moods, nutritional needs, thoughts, and cravings, all regulated by hormones. You may not have known this but your hormones depend on nutrients. If you are lacking a nutrient, it's possible your hormones may be thrown off-kilter. As a result, you can feel more sluggish, extremely emotional, have low libido, or develop hormonal acne.

Ever feel like you just can't stop crying after watching a heartfelt music video? Personally, the music video, "Happier" by Marshmello featuring Bastille has sent me into a faucet for almost an hour (cue to go to a computer and watch that video if you haven't already). It may or may not have been the hormones talking but some phases of the cycle may make you feel like you have no control over your reaction to an otherwise mundane event.

It's important to point out that some of us feel these symptoms more than others. Note that if you are on hormonal birth control or have an IUD, you may not experience the same symptoms as you would on a natural cycle. But regardless, it's always better to get in touch with how you feel throughout your cycle phases. Plus, your cycle can tell you a lot about your health status, and can reveal if you have exorbitant levels of stress, have deficiencies in essential nutrients, or suffer from a hormonal imbalance. Therefore, it's really important that you pay attention to these factors rather than ignore them.

FOOD CYCLING

Instead of letting your cycle control you, I'm going to empower you to flip that idea upside down and gain power over your cycle through food cycling. Food cycling is essentially eating the right foods for each unique phase of your cycle. It is a practice I teach in order to nutritionally get touch with your monthly cyclic rhythms, even if you are on hormonal birth control. During your monthly cycle, some days you may reach for chocolate, some days you may reach for wine, and I'm going to explain why these cravings are happening in the first place.

Take this quiz to find out if food cycling is right for you:

In the last six months, have you...

1. Gone from Positive Polly to Negative Nancy in a beat?

2. Felt irritable and had a short-fuse temper?

3. Cried easily?

4. Felt like your boobs can cut glass before your period?

5. Had a difficult time getting aroused?

6. Felt like even after a good night's rest, you want to stay in bed all day?

7. Yawned in your coworkers' faces without realizing it?

8. Had sugar cravings for just a little something sweet, after each meal?

9. Had headaches that couldn't be attributed to a hangover or dehydration?

10. Had deep or cystic pimples around your chin or cheeks that flared up during certain weeks of the month?

11. Felt like you gained weight or had difficulty losing weight, especially around your hips, thighs, and butt?

12. Felt like you couldn't stop your cravings on certain days of the month?

13. Felt anxious without being able to contribute it to something specific?

14. Felt like you were carrying around a food baby in your belly even before eating anything in the morning?

15. Felt agitated and on edge before your period?

16. Had dry or flaky skin?

17. Had noticeable cramps before your period?

18. Had an irregular or absent period?

19. Had little or no motivation to get up off the couch?

20. Had difficulty getting pregnant (after trying for six months or more)?

If you answered YES to 5 or more of these questions, go ahead and try food cycling.

Food cycling can help with:

- Mood swings and irritability
- Low libido
- Low energy
- Fatigue
- Poor sleep
- Headache
- Breast tenderness
- Uncontrollable cravings
- Premenstrual syndrome
- Hormonal acne
- Constant bloat
- Medical conditions such as polycystic ovarian syndrome (PCOS), endometriosis (abnormal growth of the tissue outside the uterus), thyroid disease, premenstrual dysphoric disorder (PMDD), and amenorrhea (the cessation of a menstrual cycle)
- Painful or heavy periods (dysmenorrhea)
- Irregular periods
- Trouble conceiving

Lots of these symptoms can be managed or even vanish through food cycling. That's the beauty of using food as medicine!

As always, it is advised to continue taking medications as prescribed by your physician and simply weave food cycling into your life. For instance, it is possible to food cycle while starting or continuing treatment with medications such as metformin or Synthroid. In fact, you may end up treating your symptoms through food cycling, but don't discontinue medication without a formal discussion with your MD.

DISCLAIMER: Please check in with your health care provider and consider food cycling once formal diagnosis/treatment options are defined. If you are having any of the above symptoms (e.g., infertility, PMDD, endometriosis, PCOS) or have a condition that needs medical attention and treatment, these need to be addressed separately and/or in combination with nutritional advice and management.

MAKING SENSE OF IT

Some of your actions could possibly be out of your control thanks to your mighty hormones. Your behaviors are actually dictated by hormonal impulses, not irrational thinking! So no need to beat yourself up if you realize you've polished off a bag of Hershey's Kisses without even noticing it!

As with every phase of your menstrual cycle, it's important to listen to your body. Don't get down on yourself if you feel extra bloated (likely just coming from water retention), or you've been MIA from your friends because you can't leave the couch. These actions are not unusual based on certain phases of your cycle. I want you to make sense of it all, which hopefully will allow you to make peace with your body and practice more self-compassion rather than getting frustrated and feeling defeated. (See Blame It on the Phase, Chapter 4.)

I want to disclose that food is just one piece of the reproductive puzzle. I do believe that food can help people heal their bodies and their minds, but it doesn't mean you should put all your eggs in one basket. That being said, use food cycling as a way to jump-start healthier eating patterns and habits, and see how far it can take you. I promise, you won't be disappointed!

BETTER PERIODS, NO MATTER THE PHASE

If you don't know where to begin, the following 10 guidelines are the perfect place for you to start. These specific strategies will allow you to start broad and then zoom into each phase of food cycling at your own pace. You can still get a better period stat by following these overall better period tips.

1. INCREASE ANTI-INFLAMMATORY FOODS

Oxidative stress not only puts a damper on our reproductive health but heightens our risk for chronic disease, illness, and even cancer. Oxidative stress can wreak havoc on our health due to the avalanche of negative and inflammatory free radical molecules, which hold the power to turn on the "harmful" DNA and turn off the "beneficial" DNA. Sometimes, we can't control oxidative stress because it can occur without us even knowing it. For example, lack of sleep, environmental pollutants, a sedentary lifestyle, alcohol, and smoking are just a few factors that can increase oxidative stress in the body. Recent studies have suggested that processed meat, such as bacon, beef, hot dogs, and luncheon meat can throw your health through the ringer, increasing inflammatory free radicals in the body and bumping up the risk for cancer and cardiovascular disease.

This is a PSA to be more mindful of added salt in your diet, which can easily lead to dehydration and unwanted bloat. Processed foods like tomato sauce, cheese, ketchup, crackers, soups, and deli meat may be filled with sodium. Plus, dressings, packaged breads, and soy sauce are shadily high in sodium. Read the nutrition labels!

However, you can swat away oxidative stress by eating more antioxidant-rich foods to help stabilize or even kill off harmful inflammation. Myriad antioxidants are obtained from food, which can reduce health risks associated with oxidative stress, one bite at a time. Phew! Thankfully, fruits and vegetables are rich sources of antioxidants, specifically those high in vitamins A, C, and E, carotenoids, and flavonoids.

In fact, jazz up your boring apple, orange, and banana game and introduce more vibrant and colorful fruits to your palate. Get inspired by unique fruits such as kiwi, papaya, star fruit, dragon fruit, and passion fruit (as displayed on the lovely cover) to help deliver an array of anti-inflammatory compounds that keep your body running like the powerful Energizer Bunny!

A greater intake of veggies has been associated with a lower incidence of oxidative stress. Aim for 5 to 13 servings of fruits and vegetables per day as recommended by the USDA. Implementing a more whole foods, plant-based diet can be your nutritional shield against chronic disease!

> If you are thinking to just go the supplement route, unfortunately supplementation with purified antioxidants have not been proven to protect against chronic disease. Let real food be your medicine!

2. ADHERE TO A MEDITERRANEAN-STYLE DIET

The Mediterranean diet can have a positive impact on your reproductive health. Research found that premenopausal women who ate a Mediterranean diet for just two months had less inflammation in the body. In fact, this style of eating can prevent diseases such as heart disease.[1]

To adopt a Mediterranean diet:

1. Simply incorporate more seafood (like salmon, mussels, and trout), vegetables, fruits, lentils, legumes, olive oil, healthy fats, whole grains, nuts, seeds, herbs, and spices.

2. Sensibly eat meat and dairy, and cut back on added sugar, refined oils, and highly processed foods.

3. Enjoy alcohol in moderation (enjoy that glass of wine, ladies).

The Mediterranean diet will inherently cause you to eat more real and whole foods coming from fruits, vegetables, whole grains, fish, and plant-based proteins. This switch may even cause weight loss

1   https://www.ncbi.nlm.nih.gov/pmc/articles/PMC2980970

because you are no longer relying on packaged foods that are often laden in sugar, sodium, and unhealthy sources of fat.

Plus, the foods on the Mediterranean diet may even help reverse diseases such as diabetes because this eating pattern can help to stabilize blood sugar. Eating more nutrient-dense, complex, whole grain carbohydrates (such as beans, buckwheat, or quinoa) will keep blood sugar levels even as you feel energized, not compromised!

If you don't want to cook an elaborate Mediterranean feast every night, you are not alone! These days, you can easily find high-quality and healthy frozen meals in the frozen section of your grocery store to help you follow a Mediterranean eating pattern. You can find frozen cauliflower rice, frozen quinoa, frozen salmon or tilapia, and voilà, you are living a Mediterranean lifestyle! Also, you can load up on no-sodium-added canned lentils or beans such as chickpeas or black beans for other plant-based protein options.

3. PUMP UP THE IRON

After your period, both your genetics and the foods you eat affect how much iron your body actually absorbs. So, while you ask mom if she's ever been anemic, make sure to be chowing down on some almonds or apricots, or have some meat roasting in the oven. Actually, researchers found that specifically high red meat consumption may protect women of childbearing age from iron deficiency.[2] When compared to consumption of several food groups (cereals, legumes, vegetables, fruits, milk and dairy products, fish, eggs, white meat, and processed meat), only red meat showed to improve iron status. Processed meat (such as deli meat and sausage) had no influence on iron status so don't load

2   https://www.ncbi.nlm.nih.gov/pubmed/24663082

up on those foods, deal? If you want to go the meat route, make sure you are buying high-quality meat from companies you trust. Though it may be pricey, it may be worth it to purchase local (when possible), grass-fed, organic beef. (Read more about iron-rich foods in Menstrual Phase Food Cycle, Part 1 on page 29.)

4. CHOOSE BETTER CARBS

Your momma was right when she said that it's always better to take it slow! And that message applies to how we pick our carbohydrates. Fiber-rich and nutrient-dense carbohydrates (like oats, beans, quinoa) are absorbed slower so your body has more time to mop up valuable vitamins and minerals. Plus, these helpful carbs keep you fuller longer so you aren't famished 15 minutes after you polish off a meal (don't you hate it when that happens?)! If you want to notice an upswing in your energy, more balanced blood sugar levels, and even a positive shift in mood, swap out fast-digesting, refined carbohydrates in your pantry like white rice and white pasta for slow-digesting brown rice and whole grain pasta.

Fiber truly is king (or should I say queen!). When it comes to hormonal balance. Bathroom talk. If you aren't going number 2 enough, estrogen can compile in the large intestine and continue to be reabsorbed again and again, leaving you with a surplus of estrogen, known as estrogen dominance. When estrogen becomes dominant in the body (either from constipation, as in this example, or because of a hormonal condition, high stress, increased alcohol consumption, or xenoestrogens, synthetic or natural chemicals imitating estrogen), it can throw everything off course, including your reproductive health.

For someone with estrogen dominance, fiber may help to even hormones out. How, you ask? Well, fiber acts as a magnet and sticks to extra estrogen hanging out in the liver and large intestine, and pushes it out of the body through poop. Cute, I know. That being said, researchers found that after just one month of taking a 10-gram wheat bran supplement in addition to eating 10 grams (about 2 teaspoons) of dietary fiber daily, estrogen was significantly reduced in the body. If there's too much estrogen in the body (particularly in endometriosis, PMS, PMDD, or PCOS), more fiber could be exactly what the doctor ordered.[3]

On the flip side, if someone is low in estrogen (typically detected by a hormonal panel or irregular or missing periods), fiber can remove too much estrogen from the body, which can negatively impact the cycle and even stop ovulation.

In order to find the perfect balance, I suggest eating moderate amounts of a wide variety of gut friendly and natural fiber-rich foods, such as fruits, vegetables, oats, lentils, quinoa, and beans to help support a balanced cycle. Remember, tailor your fiber intake to what your body and your cycle needs. (See Cut Back on High Fiber, page 152.)

Back to carb talk. Even though you may *always* crave yummy carbs, you may notice the carb cravings are particularly REAL during the menstrual and premenstrual phase. During this time, there isn't enough estrogen to power on mood-boosting chemicals like dopamine and serotonin, which is why you may find carbs extra comforting. Carbohydrates stimulate dopamine and serotonin production, which helps our brains release happy hormones and can keep our good vibes going strong.

To maintain your sanity (and your existing relationship with your significant other) don't deny yourself sustenance that makes you

---

3   https://www.sciencedirect.com/science/article/pii/S0899900797000324

feel good, just opt for slow-digesting, complex carbohydrates that are rich in belly-filling fiber. They will prevent your blood sugar from rising or dropping too quickly and will put an end to that sluggish sugar crash afterward. The best low-glycemic foods, foods that are slowly digested and absorbed, are those rich in fiber such as quinoa, whole grain pasta, brown rice, oats, lentils, beans, yams, and/or sweet potato. Don't restrict yourself from carbs from the start, just choose the right ones for your body and your brain.

5. GET ENOUGH VITAMIN D

Vitamin D is basically the quarterback of reproductive health. It has its hand in every play, from hormone-building to the development of embryos to the production of brain neurotransmitter to calcium absorption. Did you know that our bodies can't absorb calcium without vitamin D? So yes, there's a lot of pressure to get enough vitamin D.

It doesn't just stop there. Vitamin D is necessary for turning on hormones such as testosterone, progesterone, and estrogen, balancing thyroid levels and activating TSH in the pituitary gland. So, if we are deficient in vitamin D, our hormones may trudge through the mud instead of working at tip-top speed.

You can get enough vitamin D for the day through just 15 minutes of sun exposure (with SPF on too!) and from foods like fortified whole grain cereals, salmon, milk, egg yolks, and mushrooms. Vitamin D, more like vitamin Dammmmn!

6. GET PLENTY OF ZINC

An important mineral throughout the cycle, zinc doesn't get the attention it deserves! It is constantly doing maintenance on your cells to keep them pristine and healthy, and helps to keep your ovaries running in mint condition. Sufficient zinc is also needed to produce essential menstrual cycle hormones, FSH and LH, which are both vital for developing and releasing an egg during ovulation. Our bodies don't store zinc, so it's essential we get enough through our diet every day to maintain adequate hormone levels. In fact, eating zinc-rich foods like cashews, sunflower seeds, almonds, and pumpkin seeds helps produce sex hormones, like estrogen and progesterone, that are especially needed in the luteal phase. Just to cover your bases, eat enough zinc during all phases of the cycle so each phase runs steadily and smoothly. Is that a deal?

7. CONSUME HEALTHY FATS

Say, "Yes, please!" to monounsaturated fats, polyunsaturated fats, and omega-3s! It is officially time to say goodbye to that "low-fat mentality," especially if you want to better support your reproductive health. All of these healthy fats have the ability to reduce inflammation and keep your body in prime condition. Omega-3s can help combat anxiety, ward off cramps, and even help blood travel more efficiently around the body. During PMS, the uterus releases inflammatory molecules, known as prostaglandins, that could contribute to breast tenderness and bloating. If there's more inflammation in the uterus (this could be a sign of dysmenorrhea, or painful periods), it's likely you aren't going to feel your best. To help squash inflammatory pain, go for more foods rich in omega-3, like walnuts, salmon, omega-3-enriched eggs, and flaxseeds. You are going to be hearing a lot about these heart-healthy fats throughout the book, so pay attention!

8. CONSUME FOODS THAT SUPPORT GLUTATHIONE

Glutathione, a molecule containing three amino acids, is believed to offer strong antioxidant effects, enough to keep your liver running like a well-oiled machine. Because the breakdown of estrogen occurs predominantly in the liver, it's important to eat foods to help support a high-functioning liver. Glutathione may be able to flush out toxins, especially if you have extra estrogen hanging out, causing you to be estrogen dominant. Selenium, an important mineral, helps to produce more glutathione, so the more selenium, the more glutathione in the bod. Sounds like a winning combination! Eating foods rich in selenium, like Brazil nuts, cod, and shrimp, will help to keep your liver in great shape.

9. EAT MAGNESIUM-RICH FOODS

This mineral helps to achieve the perfect progesterone and estrogen balance. It also relaxes smooth muscle contractions in the uterus, which can aid in relieving period pain. Plus, magnesium can also combat pounding and painful menstrual headaches. Magnesium levels tend to go up and down throughout the cycle, which is why it's wise to eat magnesium-rich foods every day, like whole grains, flaxseeds, quinoa, and sweet potato.

10. DRINK WATER

It goes without saying that water is essential to life. Every cell in your body is dependent on water. The only downside to drinking more water is the inconvenience of having to pee more frequently, but the benefits in this situation definitely outweigh the costs. Start by drinking 1 cup of water first thing in the morning (hot, cold, with lemon, without lemon, whatever gets you to drink it!) to rehydrate your cells working hard overnight repairing and replenishing your body from head to toe.

Because the hormone progesterone can slow down digestion, it often leads to bloating and constipation. Progesterone is a natural muscle relaxant that prevents your muscles from tightening, which is crucial so your uterus can potentially foster the growth of an egg every month. Fortunately, water can help relieve the effects of progesterone's uncomfortable belly woes. Drink 9 to 13 cups of water per day, but this recommendation is different for everyone. Some people require more, some require less. Simply notice the color of your urine. If it's clear, you are drinking the right amount. If it's looking a bit darker yellow, fill up your cup of water ASAP! By scattering your water intake throughout the day (not just in one big gulp!), your body will function better, keeping your digestion going, your skin glowing, and your hormones and cells functioning just right.

To make water more interesting, add infusions to your water, such as pineapple and mint, and cucumber and basil. Don't wait any longer, go fill up that awesome refillable water bottle this instant!

FOOD CYCLING: THE BEST FOODS FOR EACH PHASE

Believe it or not, there are particular foods that are nutritionally proven to help you feel your best during each phase of your cycle.

I'll break it down into individual nutrients, and the top foods to help balance mood, feel energized, and make sure your body is working with those wild and ferocious hormones instead of against them. As a reminder, the phase lengths are approximations and your cycle length may vary, so modify and adapt the phase to your personal and unique cycle. Get your highlighters ready because you are about to get schooled!

MENSTRUAL PHASE (DAYS 1 TO 5)

FOOD CYCLE, PART 1: This is a time when your body eliminates and sheds the lining of your uterus and you have your period. Your goal is to revive your diet and add nutrients back into your body.

WHAT'S HAPPENING WITH YOUR HORMONES: As the corpus luteum, a mass of cells that produces progesterone to establish and maintain pregnancy, degenerates and no embryo is implanted (aka no bun in the oven), progesterone sharply plummets. The uterine lining (endometrium) that has been thickening and developing since your last cycle finally sheds, so you can now say hello to your period! Estrogen is at its lowest point, so the pituitary gland secretes FSH to tell the ovaries to prepare to release an egg for another round of ovulation coming right up.

FOOD + NUTRIENTS

IRON: Time to pump up the iron! Who would feel like a champ after losing about 1 teaspoon of blood every day (making some of us slightly anemic)? Certainly not me! Combating these symptoms by increasing your iron intake is key. Allow your body to take in nutrients from easy-to-absorb iron (heme iron) from animal sources like red meat, poultry, and fish. Non-animal sources of iron (nonheme) are not as easy to absorb and include plant-based, vegetarian sources like lentils, nuts, seeds, legumes, dark leafy greens, peas, and beans.

VITAMIN C: To assist in the absorption of nonheme iron, simply add vitamin C to the mix. This pairing will assist your body in absorbing iron more efficiently, and we certainly need all the iron we can get during this period of time—no pun intended! Keep lemon juice, tomatoes, bell peppers, broccoli, and citrus fruits handy for this reason. Add some lemon juice to your white beans or chickpea hummus, or throw some strawberries into your spinach salad. Not only will vitamin C aid in the absorption of iron, but it will sprinkle more inflammation-fighting antioxidants in your diet. Done and done!

VITAMIN B12: As mentioned, your body is running on low levels of estrogen and progesterone so you are more inclined to want to take a long afternoon siesta. Vitamin B12 is critical to make more red blood cells. Red blood cells carry oxygen to cells, and the more red blood cells you have, the more perked up you will be! Low levels of vitamin B12 can contribute to sleepiness, and can even cause you to feel dizzy and more nervous than usual. Pump up your vitamin B12 with some cheese, eggs, milk, fish, clams, salmon, tuna, or poultry. Because vitamin B12 is only found in animal products, if you are vegan or vegetarian, be on the lookout for fortified products that contain vitamin B12, such as alternative "alt" milks, fortified cereals, soy products, or cheese alternatives like nutritional yeast.

OMEGA-3: If you are dealing with PMS during day 1 or day 2, you are most certainly not alone! A lot of women still experience PMS (such as bloating, pain, tender breasts) in the beginning of this phase. Plus, prostaglandins, the lipid compounds responsible for pain, are coming in hot hot hot. Rather than get frustrated at your symptoms, eat foods to help combat the pain like flaxseeds, omega-3-fortified eggs, salmon, and walnuts.

ZINC: Zinc is a very important mineral during this time of the month. Zinc helps to remineralize and refresh your blood. Maintain high zinc intake during your period by eating oysters, beef, seaweed, fortified cereal, and peanut butter.

VITAMIN B: Hand over the vitamin B-rich carbs and no one gets hurt! This is NOT the phase to restrict yourself from carbs, simply choose the right ones. The best low-glycemic carbs are those rich in fiber, such as quinoa, brown rice, oats, lentils, beans, and sweet potato.

NATURAL REMEDIES: To help fight inflammation, incorporate herbs and spices such as ginger, basil, turmeric, cinnamon, garlic, parsley, and cilantro into your diet. Some proponents believe that raspberry leaf tea can reduce PMS but research is still limited.

SEED CYCLING, PHASE 1: Seed cycling is a food technique believed to regulate your cycle by rotating specific seeds in and out of your diet. I'll be going over this more in Chapter 3, Seed Cycling, but for now, if you want to seed cycle, eat 1 tablespoon of ground flaxseeds and 1 tablespoon of pumpkin seeds every day until day 14.

NUTRITIONAL NO-NOS: Reduce alcohol, spicy foods, and caffeine. High amounts of caffeine may contribute to cause heavier bleeding and heighten the risk for greater iron loss and anemia. Excessive caffeine has been shown to increase estrogen during the menstrual phase, a time when estrogen should be low.[4] To minimize hormonal disruption and imbalances, I recommend 1 to 2 cups of caffeinated beverages per day. Refined sugars from sweetened iced teas,

---

4   https://www.ncbi.nlm.nih.gov/pubmed/11591405

lemonades, and soft drinks may intensify cramps so instead, opt for unsweetened beverages like seltzers, herbal teas, or lemon water.

SO MANY FEELINGS

You may feel bloated, tired, and definitely not 100%. Iron is lost during your period so your energy dips and estrogen and progesterone are low so you definitely don't feel like a million bucks. You may be craving carbs and quick fixes (pass the bagels, please) to reduce PMS in the early days. Basically, you aren't really feelin' yourself. So, girl, your goal is to relax and recover RIGHT NOW!

FATIGUE: It's okay to be sleepy, especially due to the drop in circulating estrogen and progesterone. Therefore, it may not be best to take on a grueling spin class or a crazy new home project. Make time for yoga, walking, and light stretching, which is OK! We aren't meant to be "on" every day of the month, and this 100% holds true during this phase. Just take it slow.

CRAVINGS: You may crave warm foods, such as stews, soups, or warm stir-fries that help you feel cozy. Lean into these soothing options to get re-energized, nourished, and reinvigorated for the upcoming phase of the cycle.

CRAMPS: Especially during the first few days of our period, cramps may come in strong. The uterus has to contract in order to release the uterine lining, so it's no mystery why we may have throbbing pain. As the lining gets ready to be released in the menstrual phase, some also feel this discomfort in the late luteal phase as well. Hold on for the ride, ladies!

FOLLICULAR PHASE (DAYS 6 TO 11)

The follicular phase technically begins the first day of your period and ends when you begin ovulation. For the purpose of food cycling, the follicular phase eating plan begins once your period ends. This will help keep food and nutrient guidelines and suggestions as specific as possible.

FOOD CYCLE, PART 2: This is a time when estrogen starts to increase as your body prepares to release a mature follicle (egg) during ovulation. Your goal is to eat a wholesome, well-rounded diet with colorful nutrients.

WHAT'S HAPPENING WITH YOUR HORMONES: The body is preparing for ovulation. Progesterone and estrogen are low at the start of this phase, which triggers the pituitary gland to wake up FSH. FSH stimulates the growth of maturing egg follicles, which are fluid-filled sacs in the ovary containing an egg. Several egg follicles expand but only one mature egg is released during ovulation (unless you have twins on your hands, but that's another story). The dominant follicle prompts estrogen to rise at the end of the phase, with the goal of preparing the uterus to safely support a pregnancy. The phase ends when LH increases sharply, which stimulates ovulation, the release of the mature egg with hopes of fertilization. As for the other hormones, testosterone starts to rise at the tail end of the phase while progesterone remains low.

FOOD + NUTRIENTS

PHYTOESTROGEN FOODS: Keep your rising estrogen levels stable by eating foods that help regulate and support estrogen. Start with flaxseeds and pumpkin seeds, both key players if you want to start seed cycling (see Chapter 3). Other foods that are high in phytoestrogens are soybeans, hummus, berries, grains, spinach, garlic, fennel, and alfalfa sprouts.

FIBER: Fiber is a type of carbohydrate that the body craves during this phase to keep estrogen balanced and to promote regularity. Examples of fiber-rich foods are oats, brown rice, lentils, beans, berries, nuts, seeds, and apples.

ANTIOXIDANT-RICH FOODS: Colorful foods all the way! Aim for foods overflowing in antioxidants (see page 92), like vitamins A, C, and E. They will not only help nourish the growing follicle during ovulation but will also reduce harmful oxidative stress in the body. Research found that high levels of oxidative stress in the body were correlated to high estrogen typically seen before ovulation.[5] In fact, you may even lose vitamin C right before ovulation so it's very important to load up. Therefore, sprinkle your plate with colorful and vibrant foods to kick unwelcome stress and oxidation to the curb, such as strawberries, broccoli, sweet potatoes, carrots, and citrus fruits.

SPICY FOODS: Time to spice up your life! Spicy foods may have the ability to decrease oxidative stress and lessen inflammation–the less inflammation around our lady parts, the better! Eat some spicy foods coming from capsaicin, the active compound of chili, jalapeño, and cayenne peppers. In animal studies, capsaicin-rich diets may reduce the risk for heart disease, diabetes, and hypertension. Although future clinical studies are needed to establish a protocol tolerable for humans, capsaicin can potentially improve metabolic, vascular, and circulatory health. If you are sensitive to spicy foods or experience stomach discomfort after eating spicy foods, it's probably best not to go full throttle with the spicy fare. Simply tailor

---

5   https://www.ncbi.nlm.nih.gov/pmc/articles/PMC2950793/#bib38

your food choices according to your spice tolerance and flavor preferences.

FERMENTED FOODS: If you've had an upset belly during menstruation due to low hormone levels, it's time to repair it during this phase with gut-healing foods. Support gut balance and good bacteria restoration with probiotic-rich foods like yogurt and kefir, prebiotic-rich foods like onions, bananas, and garlic, and fermented foods such as pickled veggies, sauerkraut, and kimchi.

LIVER "DETOX" FOODS: Sulfur-rich foods, such as Brussels sprouts, cabbage, cauliflower, and broccoli, contain indoles, compounds that have protective effects on the liver. These vegetables will help metabolize excess estrogen in the liver if there is too much hanging out.

HEALTHY FAT: It's beneficial to eat more healthy fat leading up to ovulation because it ensures your body has enough energy to develop and release a healthy follicle. Because your appetite is relatively low around ovulation due to the anorectic (appetite-suppressing) effects of estrogen, eating healthy fats will secure healthy hormone production needed to fuel and protect the cycle. Opt for mono- and polyunsaturated fats, such as nuts, seeds, olive oil, and avocado, to help promote stellar reproductive health and ovulation.

ZINC: Aim for zinc from yummy sources like avocado, eggs, nuts, seeds, whole grains, and chickpeas to help support egg development during this phase.

ALCOHOL: Although the research remains a bit murky, studies have shown that alcohol can mess with estrogen metabolism in the liver. Both alcohol and estrogen rely on the liver for metabolism. When both alcohol and estrogen are thrown into the mix, estrogen metabolism takes a backseat and alcohol gets flushed and metabolized first. This subsequently can lead to estrogen buildup in the blood. In studies, alcohol consumption led to estrogen remaining in the blood after an estrogen patch was given to postmenopausal women, and alcohol increased estrogen levels from oral contraceptives in premenopausal women.[6, 7] Therefore, it may be wise to drink alcohol in moderation during this phase to prevent estrogen from compounding in the body and to keep hormones balanced!

FERTILITY-BOOSTING FOODS: Focus on eating a wide variety of fertility-boosting foods, especially before ovulation. See Chapter 10 for fertility-boosting foods you should be eating *all month long*!

SO MANY FEELINGS

You are glowing, lady! Rising estrogen promotes feel-good hormones. As estrogen levels creep up, so does energy and confidence, giving you a natural high! Your libido starts to rebuild, thanks to estrogen and testosterone. Climbing levels of estrogen may slightly suppress the appetite at the end of the phase, so it's no wonder you aren't as focused on food as you normally are.

IMPROVED ENERGY: Although you may have felt sluggish during menstruation because hormones were at their lowest point, your mood and brain power begin to improve as estrogen and testosterone start to rise.

CHANGING APPETITE: In the beginning, your hunger may be slightly higher than it was during the menstrual phase but not as high as it will be in the luteal phase when progesterone spills in. When estrogen sharply soars at the end of the follicular phase, there's a noticeable

6   https://www.ncbi.nlm.nih.gov/pubmed/7750592
7   https://www.ncbi.nlm.nih.gov/pubmed/10397281

dip in food intake. That's because sexual motivation and desire take over as the fertility window (ovulation) gets closer and closer!

SEXY AF: Rising testosterone helps to stimulates your libido, which starts to make you feel sexy as you get ready for ovulation. Ooh la la!

OVULATION OR OVULATORY PHASE (DAYS 12 TO 14, HALFWAY POINT)

FOOD CYCLE, PART 3: This is a time when your body releases an egg and hormones have boosted. Your goal is to choose high-quality nutrition over high-quantity nutrition.

WHAT'S HAPPENING WITH YOUR HORMONES: FSH has fallen and high estrogen triggers the sharp spike of LH from the pituitary gland, known as the LH surge. The LH surge prompts the follicle to release the egg, which travels to the fallopian tube, where it can be fertilized by sperm for 24 to 72 hours. High levels of estrogen promote your cervix to release sticky mucus, helping to protect and trap any sperm that's swimming to meet the egg. Note, sperm can last up to five days in the uterus so technically, it can enter you even before ovulation, making fertilization possible. Just a friendly reminder for those who aren't looking to get pregnant!

Estrogen levels that have remained high from the follicular phase finally peak during ovulation, around days 12 to 14. Testosterone also peaks during ovulation thanks to the surge in LH. Progesterone starts to gradually increase thanks to the development of the corpus luteum.

FOOD + NUTRIENTS

FIBER: Maintaining a healthy gut microbiome is pivotal in striking the right hormonal balance. Believe it or not, gut bacteria decides the levels of hormones needed to achieve the perfect harmony between estrogen and progesterone. In order to find that sweet spot during this phase (and remember, you may not be starving the way you typically are), opt for less-filling fiber-rich foods like quinoa, berries, couscous, and farro.

LIVER "DETOX" FOODS: To keep your liver shining bright like a diamond, increase glutathione by eating sulfur-rich foods like kale, cauliflower, Brussels sprouts, and mustard greens. Antioxidant-rich raspberries, strawberries, and bell peppers also boost glutathione. Or, get glutathione directly from spinach, avocado, and asparagus. Finally, add more allium-rich vegetables, such as onions, garlic, and shallots, which help your liver run smoothly. Tip: Cooking may reduce the bioavailability and levels of glutathione so it's best to eat those foods raw when possible.

ZINC: Known to facilitate healthy ovulation, zinc is a powerful antioxidant that helps support high-quality eggs. Regardless if you are looking to get pregnant or not, zinc helps your cells stay fresh and red-carpet ready at all times. Zinc-rich sources include pumpkin seeds, oats, quinoa, figs, and whole grains.

MAGNESIUM: Get ahead of the inevitable magnesium dip during ovulation and add hempseed, flaxseed, tofu, almonds, quinoa, sorghum, and barley into your life! Ensuring that you eat enough magnesium during this phase can prevent any magnesium deficiencies.

PROTEIN: If you feel like maximizing your time at the gym during this phase, you are not alone! High level of testosterone will push you toward putting more OOMPH into your workouts. Supply your body with adequate protein during this time to properly repair and rebuild muscle tissue post workout. Think lean cuts of meat and poultry, fish, eggs, Greek yogurt, and nuts. Because you may not be feeling especially hungry during this phase, these protein-rich foods fuel your body and keep energy levels sustained, regardless if you get a workout in or not.

ALCOHOL: Researchers believe estrogen may alter dopamine levels, thus reinforcing the rewarding effects of alcohol and causing women to want to drink more during ovulation when estrogen is high.[8] Therefore, alcohol feels much more exciting and rewarding during this phase, and we are more susceptible to abuse it. Research also suggests that women more vulnerable to addiction may be even more likely to seek out the pleasurable and euphoric effects associated with alcohol consumption during this phase.[9] So, keep an eye out for how alcohol influences you before you reach for another glass of pinot!

SO MANY FEELINGS

You are feeling like the king (or should I say queen) of the world! High energy, more confidence, positive vibes all around. Honey, you are glowing! As far as your hunger, estrogen's appetite-suppressing effects puts a pause on your love for pizza and pasta as you become more interested in getting it on! Cue Marvin Gaye please...

STRUT GF! Estrogen is elevated and testosterone has peaked. You feel even more sexy, even more assertive, and unapologetically confident. Can't stop, won't stop!

8   https://journals.plos.org/plosone/article?id=10.1371/journal.pone.0187698
9   Ibid.

CONFUSION DOWN UNDER: Um, what's that? Don't be alarmed, it's just your cervical mucus saying hello. You may notice a change in your vaginal discharge, as it becomes clear and stretchy, like raw egg whites during this phase. No need to panic, it's natural, and a good sign of reproductive health!

CRAVINGS: Thanks to both estrogen and testosterone coming to the party, sexual desire peaks and women shift their behaviors from feeding and foraging to wanting sex. As the fertility window opens, this hormonal trade-off has been instrumental, not to mention necessary, in keeping the mammalian species alive. Progesterone, known to boost appetite, is low during ovulation because sex hormones are designed to manipulate and suppress hunger when conception is possible. Scientists believe that women have a lower threshold for satiety (meaning you get fuller faster) during the fertile window to open up more time to engage in mating.[10] Therefore, opt for higher-quality foods over higher-quantity so you have plenty of time for hanky-panky.

I LIKE TO MOVE IT MOVE IT: Find those high-intensity interval training (HIIT) workouts like spin classes, CrossFit, and boot camp! High levels of testosterone will help you put more power into your workouts and may even cause you to unexpectedly grunt during that final rep of weights!

LUTEAL/PREMENSTRUAL PHASE (DAYS 15 TO 28)

FOOD CYCLE, PART 4: This is a time when your body preps for your next period by building and thickening the uterine lining. Or maybe you've become pregnant. Either way, your goal is to hold on for the ride.

---

10   https://www.ncbi.nlm.nih.gov/pubmed/28202355

WHAT'S HAPPENING WITH YOUR HORMONES: The corpus luteum pumps out high amounts of progesterone (and some estrogen) to help build and thicken the uterine lining to prepare for potential pregnancy. Right now, there is basically a progesterone party going on in the body. Testosterone has left the building, and estrogen is playing second fiddle to the surge of progesterone. Hormones like LH and FSH are low. If the egg doesn't become fertilized by sperm, the corpus luteum disintegrates and breaks down, and so does the uterine lining, causing progesterone and estrogen to decline, and some experience PMS. By the end, the progesterone drop will prompt day 1 of menstruation as you begin your cycle again.

Fun fact: The luteal phase is the most definitive of the phases. That's because it doesn't vary, it always occurs from ovulation until the first day of menses. Period, end of story.

FOOD + NUTRIENTS

WATER: Annoying and obvious tip, but drinking enough water is extremely necessary to combat bloat. After a hibachi dinner or a Chipotle burrito, it's likely you may feel bloated, but in this phase, you don't necessarily have to eat too much sodium to feel like a balloon. That's because elevated estrogen and progesterone levels cause us to retain more water. Studies have found that progesterone and estrogen may disrupt fluid and sodium regulation in the body.[11] So, it's no wonder the thought of putting on your "skinny" jeans make you want to scream. Thank goodness for trendy stretchy track pants!

---

11   https://www.ncbi.nlm.nih.gov/pmc/articles/PMC2849969

NATURAL SUGARS: Work with your expected low energy and think ahead to stock up on natural sweets, like dark chocolate, peanut butter, yogurt, honey, fresh or dried fruit, or smoothies. These natural sweets will give your brain a quick energy boost while putting a smile on your face. See Chapter 4, Blame It on the Phase, for more information.

SEED CYCLING, PHASE 2: Swap out phase 1 seeds and swap in 1 tablespoon of sunflower seeds and 1 tablespoon of sesame seeds per day for days 15 to 28 on Phase 2. Please read Chapter 3.

- Vitamin D: See page 82.
- Omega-3: See page 81.
- Magnesium: See page 86.
- B vitamins: See page 80.

NATURAL REMEDIES: Essential oils may help lessen cramps, especially lavender, sage, and marjoram. Women who used cream with these oils (instead of placebo-controlled oils) felt relief in the intensity and duration of cramps.[12] To help fight inflammation, incorporate herbs and spices into your diet such as ginger, basil, turmeric, cinnamon, garlic, parsley, and cilantro. Agnus castus fruit extract, also known as chasteberry, may be able to relieve PMS symptoms but research is mixed.[13]

SO MANY FEELINGS

This phase requires a higher demand of energy coming from nutrients and food to help rebuild the uterine lining. You will be your hungriest, as you crave more fat and more carbs. You'll have

---

12   https://obgyn.onlinelibrary.wiley.com/doi/full/10.1111/j.1447-0756.2011.01802.x#acces sDenialLayout
13   https://www.ncbi.nlm.nih.gov/pubmed/11159568

fewer feel-good hormones, more anxiety, more fatigue, and more bloating, and you'll probably think the couch has never looked more appealing. PMS may kick in toward the latter end of the phase. Yup, that means cramps, belly woes, difficulty sleeping, headaches, and more *hangry* moments. Check out how to nutritionally manage PMS in Chapter 5.

THE BLOATING IS REAL: Keep water handy during this phase to avoid feeling like a balloon! When estrogen and progesterone levels are higher, our bodies tend to hold onto more water. Retaining water is your body's way of preventing us from becoming dehydrated, which is albeit uncomfortable, is actually very important in maintaining homeostasis. Bonus, progesterone (that is in high gear) can slow down the digestive tract, further contributing to bloat. To ease the bloat, drink more fluids to reduce salt retention and to help promote bathroom regularity. Opt for soothing teas such as peppermint, spearmint, or ginger tea to both ease inflammation and hydrate. I suggest purchasing a 32-ounce water bottle to maintain fluid balance in order to successfully button your pants!

SWEET TEMPTATIONS: Sweet cravings and increased appetite are especially present, and as a result, women take in more calories and have a stronger desire for high-fat foods and higher-complex carbohydrates during this time. This may be related to the synthesis of beta-endorphins, an endorphin known to suppress pain, which can in turn stimulate the appetite.[14]

There are two specific times during the luteal phase when you may feel sugar cravings are especially pronounced. The first is during the beginning of the luteal phase, before progesterone kicks in (think days 15 to 18) and the second is when estrogen dips near

---

14 https://www.jstor.org/stable/29540529

the end of the luteal phase (think days 25 to 28). But don't worry, these strong sugar cravings and even heightened emotions, like anxiety or stress, are typical.

LOW SEXUAL DESIRE: Progesterone has the ability to not only increase your food intake by fighting against estrogen's appetite-suppressing effects, but it can also smash your libido. Plus, testosterone is low during this phase, which inherently suppresses your sexual desire. So, if you aren't in the mood for doing the deed, tell your partner it's not them, it's the hormones!

CHARITABLE: The luteal phase ignites a more social female, looking to foster and build relationships. A study found that women are more inclined to give gifts to loved ones and donate more money and time to charity during the luteal phase.[15] This phase motivates women to nurture social alliances, so instead of curling up on the couch solo, go hang with your gal pals!

ANXIETY OVERLOAD: Women with higher average progesterone levels across their cycle reported higher levels of anxiety than women with lower progesterone.[16] Although progesterone is an antianxiety hormone, it's possibly that too much progesterone can send cortisol and stress into overdrive. In addition to higher anxiety, it's possible to be more stressed in the luteal phase compared to the follicular phase because elevated hormones may amplify cortisol activity.[17] If this sounds like you, keep chamomile tea, essential oils like lavender, as well as warm foods like soups or stews handy to calm your firing nerves.

---

15   https://www.sciencedirect.com/science/article/abs/pii/S014829631730437X
16   https://www.ncbi.nlm.nih.gov/pubmed/29673619
17   https://www.ncbi.nlm.nih.gov/pubmed/29605399

SEED CYCLING

If you have no idea what seed cycling is, you are not alone. Sometimes referred to as seed rotation, seed cycling means swapping seeds in and out of your diet, depending on the day of your cycle. Seed cycling is a hot and trendy topic at the moment, touted to help you achieve a better, healthier, and more balanced cycle.

There are four seeds to eat during seed cycling to gain special nutritional perks: flaxseeds, pumpkin seeds, sesame seeds, and sunflower seeds. And there is a certain protocol to eating them. For example, you eat flaxseeds and pumpkin seeds every day during the first half of your cycle (days 1 to 14). During the second half (days 15 to 28), you swap out those seeds and replace them with sesame seeds and sunflower seeds. Please note that seed cycling is based off a 28-day monthly cycle.

Before I go any further about seed cycling, let me be clear. There has been research on the benefits of eating specific seeds to nutritionally support *your hormones* but not on the connection between the suggested seed cycling protocol and hormonal balance.

That is why I simply encourage *eating more seeds* for the sole reason that seeds are actually extremely healthy and very natural. Think of seed cycling as a nudge in the right direction to eat more real food in general that is rich in essential vitamins and minerals.

Seed cycling could be right for those with a predictable cycle, those with a hormonal imbalance, and those on birth control. Seed cycling may ease PMS, relieve symptoms related to PCOS, lessen pain from endometriosis, reduce dysmenorrhea, combat amenorrhea, and help fight off fatigue, sleep disturbances, irregular cycles, hormonal-related acne, and more.

Remember, hormones are meant to go up and down throughout the cycle. Certain seeds could mess with the natural hormonal fluctuations throughout the cycle, so it's important you check with your medical professional to know what hormones you need to pay extra attention to.

From what I've seen in my practice, seed cycling is not particularly dangerous and does not pose any major health risk. I've seen how it can help people feel better about regulating their hormones and reduce PMS, but *I do not think it is the magical cure-all.*

HORMONAL BALANCE FOR ALL

Guess what does an incredible job at maintaining our delicate hormonal equilibrium? Our organs! The kidneys, liver, and intestines work hard 24/7 to maintain hormonal balance. However, this filtering system can get backed up if we are exposed to high amounts of organ and endocrine disruptors (coming from toxins, metals, plastics), constantly feel stressed (causing our sympathetic nervous system to spill out fight-or-flight hormones and cortisol), aren't sleeping enough, and are omitting specific nutrients from our diets.

If our organs are working overtime, we may notice jarring symptoms such as PMS, acne, moodiness, and fatigue. Seeds are thought to bring your organs back to speed to handle the hormonal load. Think of the seeds as Santa's little helpers, who assist with the job when needed. Basically, eating more seeds can help the body recalibrate, which is why I support the notion of sprinkling more seeds into your diet. I'll help you understand what we currently know about seed cycling and how it can potentially help you take control of your menstrual health.

The Seed Cycling Cycle

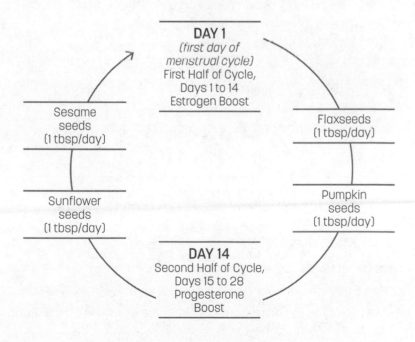

These are recommendations based on an average 28-day cycle:

FIRST HALF, DAYS 1 TO 14, or from new moon to full moon if you don't have your period or it is irregular. (You can easily Google what moon it is right now.)

1 tablespoon per day of ground flaxseeds

1 tablespoon per day of pumpkin seeds (optional to grind)

SECOND HALF, DAYS 15 TO 28, or from full moon to new moon if you don't have your period or it is irregular.

1 tablespoon per day of sunflower seeds (optional to grind)

1 tablespoon per day of sesame seeds (optional to grind)

Women's cycles can be linked up with the rhythms of the moon. Women with irregular cycles or with cycles too short or too long may be able to follow the rhythms of the lunar cycle to sync up with their cycle. For instance, at the new moon, start with phase 1 of seed cycling and switch to phase 2 at the full moon. It may be a little bit woo-woo to do this, but it's worth a shot!

FLAXSEEDS, PHASE 1

GOAL: BOOST AND BALANCE ESTROGEN

The goal in eating flaxseeds is to strike the perfect estrogen balance in this phase. We want to make enough estrogen during this phase to help rebuild the uterine lining, but not land ourselves in a state of estrogen dominance. If there's too much estrogen in the body, we may experience PMS, bloating, and breast tenderness. No thanks!

FLAXSEEDS 101

Shown to mimic and impact estrogen metabolism, flaxseeds are one of the richest sources of lignans and isoflavones, a group of plant nutrients known as phytoestrogens. Flaxseeds may protect us from estrogen dominance in the body. If there is a spillover of estrogen in the body, lignans can help sweep excess estrogen out. This can be very helpful for those with PMS, PCOS, thyroid dysfunction, lack of ovulation, irregular periods, or a history of breast cancer.

> Those with breast cancer or a history of breast cancer are advised to avoid significant phytoestrogen intake (like flaxseeds) including but not limited to black cohosh, red clover, evening primrose oil (or supplements that contain these items), and excessive dietary soy intake. Therefore, please consult your MD before you decide to incorporate flaxseeds into your daily routine.

To achieve estrogen balance, researchers believe the lignans in flaxseeds can change estrogen behavior. Based on what the body needs, lignans can either block or encourage estrogen absorption, so they behave in multiple ways depending on the body's condition.[18, 19] Lignans' impact on estrogen is still a very hot topic and more research is brewing.

18   https://www.ncbi.nlm.nih.gov/pmc/articles/PMC4375225
19   https://www.ncbi.nlm.nih.gov/pubmed/19921254

WHAT THE RESEARCH SAYS

RESTORE HORMONAL BALANCE

- Flaxseeds can stop the conversion of the sex hormone androgens (such as testosterone) to estrogen, which helps to keep estrogen levels low.[20, 21]

- Taking 25 grams (~4 tablespoons) of ground flaxseeds/day significantly reduced estrogen activity in postmenopausal women.[22]

- Lignans can stimulate a hormone made in the liver called sex hormone binding globulin (SHBG), that decreased the circulation and activity of estrogen, testosterone, and dihydro-testosterone.[23, 24] This may be helpful in those with PCOS.

- Ground flaxseeds also contain a high amount of fiber (the most of all the seeds involved in seed cycling), which can help remove excess estrogen from the body.

HELP WITH OVULATION

In a small study, regularly cycling women were monitored for three months while eating a typical omnivorous, low-fiber diet. They were then monitored for another three months while eating the same diet, but now supplemented with ground flaxseed. Women taking *1 tablespoon of ground flaxseed daily resulted in more months with ovulation* when compared to the control diet without ground flaxseed.[25] Reasons why someone can have anovulatory cycles (cycles without ovulation) include diminished ovarian reserve, primary ovarian insufficiency, age, or PCOS.

20   https://www.ncbi.nlm.nih.gov/pubmed/19921254
21   https://www.ncbi.nlm.nih.gov/pubmed/8382517
22   https://academic.oup.com/ajcn/article/79/2/318/4690098
23   https://www.ncbi.nlm.nih.gov/pubmed/8681458
24   https://www.ncbi.nlm.nih.gov/pubmed/12270221
25   https://academic.oup.com/jcem/article-abstract/77/5/1215/2649961?redirectedFrom=fulltext

REDUCE PMS AND INFLAMMATION

Flaxseeds have omega-3 fatty acids, an inflammation fighter. Our actual period, starting on day 1, is in and of itself an inflammatory process. Therefore, flaxseeds may stand up to PMS-related pain and inflammation. Flaxseeds have also been shown to reduce C-reactive protein, a protein produced by the liver when there is inflammation detected in the body.[26, 27]

TRACY'S TAKEAWAYS

Flaxseeds offer anti-inflammatory and fiber-filled benefits, may increase ovulation, and may help detoxify the body of excess estrogen when needed. Talk about a functional food!

PUMPKIN SEEDS, PHASE 1

GOAL: BOOST AND BALANCE ESTROGEN

Pumpkin seeds are high in nutrients like anti-inflammatory omega-3 and omega-6 fatty acids and have similar lignans as found in flaxseeds.

WHAT THE RESEARCH SAYS

MENOPAUSE SYMPTOMS

Supplementing with pumpkin seed oil minimizes menopausal symptoms such as hot flashes, headaches, and joint pain.[28]

26 https://www.sciencedirect.com/science/article/pii/S0271531798001006
27 https://www.ncbi.nlm.nih.gov/pubmed/18502107
28 https://www.ncbi.nlm.nih.gov/pubmed/21545273

REDUCE ESTROGEN

Eating pumpkin seeds has been shown to reduce excess estrogen as well as decrease the risk of estrogen-receptive positive breast cancer by 12% in postmenopausal women.[29]

TRACY'S TAKEAWAYS

Pumpkin seed benefits are promising in alleviating PMS symptoms, thanks to the inflammation-fighting and health-boosting powers of nutrients like magnesium and zinc. See Chapter 5, Premenstrual Disorders for more on magnesium and zinc benefits.

SUNFLOWER SEEDS, PHASE 2

GOAL: BOOST AND BALANCE PROGESTERONE

The next phase focuses on eating seeds to boost progesterone. Progesterone helps further thicken the uterine lining and prepare it for a potential pregnancy each month. Sunflower seeds are rich sources of linoleic acid, a calming omega-6 fatty acid that may help to relax muscles. Sunflower seeds can reduce pain and bloating stemming from menstrual cramps. They are also rich in vitamins B1 and B6 and magnesium, all of which can help lessen PMS.

---

29   https://www.ncbi.nlm.nih.gov/pubmed/22591208

WHAT THE RESEARCH SAYS

SELENIUM POWER

Sunflower seeds are made up of powerful antioxidants like selenium that help support the reproductive system and the metabolism of thyroid hormones.[30] Just 2 teaspoons of sunflower seeds provide women 31% of the recommended daily allowance (RDA) of selenium.

PROGESTERONE BOOST

In research, vitamin E helps to increase progesterone, and sunflower seeds are excellent sources of vitamin E.

ESTROGEN REDUCER

Eating sunflower seeds has been shown to remove excess estrogen in the body.[31]

TRACY'S TAKEAWAYS

1. Though large-scale human studies on the benefits of sunflower seeds on the menstrual cycle are lacking, there are many perks to adding sunflower seeds to the diet to deliver helpful omega-6s, zinc, selenium, vitamin E, and a ton of B vitamins. Plus, 2 tablespoons of sunflower seeds provide a good source of iron, which lots of women tend to be low in, especially if they experience heavy blood loss during their period.

2. It's typical to feel blue during the luteal phase, because the mood-boosting neurotransmitter serotonin is out of the office. However, the B vitamins in sunflower seeds have the ability to

30   https://www.ncbi.nlm.nih.gov/pmc/articles/PMC5666889
31   https://www.ncbi.nlm.nih.gov/pubmed/22591208

boost mood and help to reduce anxiety during this cloudy phase. See Chapter 5, Premenstrual Disorders, for more on reducing PMS symptoms.

SESAME SEEDS, PHASE 2

GOAL: BOOST AND BALANCE PROGESTERONE

Just like the other seeds, sesame seeds also contain hormone-regulating lignans, anti-inflammatory essential fatty acids, and phytoestrogens. Compared to the other seeds, sesame seeds are the highest in zinc, which has been found to squash period pain.[32]

Just like the sunflower seed, sesame seeds are excellent sources of linoleic acid, providing a hefty dose of heart-healthy and inflammation-fighting omega-6s. Make sure to get enough vitamin B, zinc, and magnesium to transform the nutrients in sesame seeds into usable brain-healthy compounds such as DHA and EPA. Next time, sprinkle some sesame seeds on top of your oats or throw a bunch on your morning scrambled eggs!

WHAT THE RESEARCH SAYS

REDUCE EXCESS ESTROGEN

SHBG can increase significantly after eating 7 tablespoons of powdered ground sesame seeds for five weeks, which may help remove excess estrogen in the body.[33]

---

32   https://www.ncbi.nlm.nih.gov/pubmed/26132140
33   https://academic.oup.com/jn/article/136/5/1270/4669984

REDUCE EXCESS ANDROGENS

Sex hormone androgens significantly decreased after eating 7 tablespoons of ground sesame seeds for five weeks. Sesame seeds may be helpful for those with high levels of androgens, specifically in PCOS.[34]

Evening Primrose Oil

Evening primrose oil is an optional add-on to phase 2. Evening primrose oil is known as gamma linolenic acid (GLA), which is rich in omega-6s. Found to fight inflammation, GLA from food sources may stop the growth of inflamed endometrial tissue.[35] The best food sources of GLA are found in hemp seeds, whole grains, and Ezekiel bread.

There is still not enough evidence to support the use of evening primrose oil due to its potentially dangerous side effects, especially in those with a heart condition or those taking heart meds. Alternative medicine is not a substitute for standard medical care, so keep that in mind!

REVIVE THE PERIOD

Roughly 4 tablespoons of ground sesame seeds taken for seven days help to jump-start menstruation and treat oligomenorrhea, or infrequent menstruation.[36]

---

34   https://academic.oup.com/jn/article/136/5/1270/4669984
35   https://www.ncbi.nlm.nih.gov/pubmed/17168669
36   http://emedicalj.com/en/articles/20393.html

PROGESTERONE PARTY

Sesame seeds are filled to the brim with zinc, which may help boost progesterone. Research has found progesterone and zinc work together in achieving hormonal balance.

ANTI-INFLAMMATORY PROPERTIES

Sesame seeds are truly fantastic for your health! They prevent amazing antioxidants, like vitamin E and gamma-tocopherol, from breaking down in the body so they can continue working their healing magic. These antioxidants are especially important in the luteal phase when your period (aka inflammation) is just around the corner. Think of sesame seeds like an all-star soccer goalie who's defending and protecting your health with all their might!

TRACY'S TAKEAWAYS

While there is limited evidence sesame seeds can significantly manipulate hormonal balance, they are a healthy addition to your diet. Nutritious benefits to the body include reduced inflammation and a boost of antioxidants coming from zinc and vitamin E.

THE VERDICT

If you see the upsides in trying seed cycling, go for it! Try seed cycling for at least three to four months in order to take note of any profound differences. Track any symptoms you have before seed cycling (acne, bloating, cramps) and afterward to see any remarkable changes.

Seed cycling isn't an exact science, *clearly*, but we can all benefit from the bountiful omega-3, omega-6, antioxidants, vitamins, and minerals found in seeds! The specific vitamins and minerals in the seeds (such as zinc, magnesium, vitamin E, and vitamin B1) *have* been well researched as tools to help mitigate painful period symptoms. Remember, seed cycling might not be able to completely rebalance your hormonal system like you may have hoped but *it can absolutely support your journey* toward a healthier diet. And who doesn't want to sprinkle their diets with the unique flavor profiles and crunchy goodness coming from seeds? Remember the power of standing behind real food!

GENERAL SEED CYCLING GUIDELINES + OTHER USEFUL SEED TIPS

1. Be sure to use raw, organic seeds when possible. Commercial roasted nuts are not advised.

2. If you are allergic to seeds, don't eat them!

3. If you've never consumed seeds before, start slowly and work your way up to 2 tablespoons per day to prevent abdominal discomfort, bloating, and diarrhea.

4. Drink at least 8 to 16 ounces of water with a meal containing seeds to promote bowel regularity.

5. If seeds are upsetting your stomach, try soaking them in warm water for 8 to 10 hours to increase their digestibility. Plus, soaking can reduce phytic acid and boost absorption of nutrients.

6. Sprouted seeds may be easier for some folks to digest (flaxseeds do not need to be soaked or sprouted). If it's still painful, stop.

7. Buy fresh flaxseeds and grind. Flaxseeds must be ground just before eating to reduce spoilage and promote absorption.

8. Buy whole, dry, golden-yellow, or brown flaxseeds instead of already ground powder to ensure highest nutritional quality. When grinding seeds, use a coffee or spice grinder. Don't grind all at once (only a three- or four-day supply at a time or even right before eating) because the seeds may become rancid and oxidize after grinding.

9. Store all seeds in a glass jar (I love my mason jars!) with a tight seal and keep in the refrigerator.

10. The strongest evidence to help restore your period and your ovulation is adding 1 to 2 tablespoons of ground flaxseeds daily to your diet.

11. You can start seed cycling on any day of your cycle, just be sure to choose the right seeds for that phase.

12. If you want more than just the seeds, some proponents suggest adding a combo of EPA and DHA fish oil (1,500 milligrams per day) during phase 1 and evening primrose oil to phase 2. The dose for EPA is 500 to 6,000mg one to four times daily for up to 10 months. Start with the smallest dose possible and increase as needed to relieve symptoms. Talk to your doctor about the best regimen for you.

13. You can still seed cycle if you have PMS, PMDD, PCOS, endometriosis, hypo/hyperthyroid, Hashimoto's disease, Graves' disease, or amenorrhea, or are in menopause, on birth control, or on other hormonal contraceptives.

14. If you are inspired to eat other seeds such as hemp, chia, or watermelon seeds to obtain similar health benefits of seed cycling seeds such as omega-3, zinc, folate, iron, and magnesium, go for it!

15. Good and healthy bacteria is necessary to break down the seeds in the gut so it's super important to maintain a healthy microbiome. A new area of research is exploring how a collection of genes, bacteria, and enzymes, known as the estrobolome, is responsible for regulating and breaking down estrogen in the gut. By getting plenty of probiotics in food to power up your internal ecosystem, you'll be able to keep those hormone levels in check! See Probiotics on page 91.

16. Most of the research has been done on eating seeds for longer than two weeks, so if you want to keep eating a particular seed because it is helping your symptoms, there's no need to take it out after two weeks.

17. If eating seeds causes you to stress out for any reason, don't do it. Please!

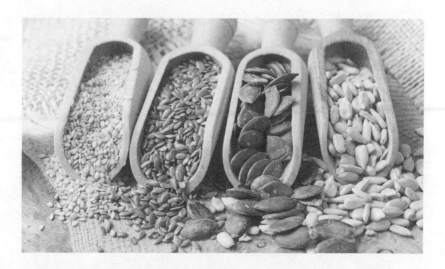

Ideas for eating more seeds:

- Add them to yogurt, overnight oats, and chia seed pudding oatmeal.
- Sprinkle sesame seeds on ground tahini.
- Make a flaxseed pudding with Greek yogurt.
- Toss them on a salad.
- Sneak them into wraps.
- Sprinkle some on your sweet potato.
- Bake some into muffins.
- Make a pumpkin bread.
- Sprinkle some in pancake or waffle batter.
- Hide them in homemade cookies.
- Make a fresh seed butter to spread on apples.
- Make a pumpkin seed pesto with bean-based pasta.
- Add seeds into your morning smoothie.

Seed Nutrient Comparison

NUTRIENT	FLAXSEEDS	PUMPKIN SEEDS	SUNFLOWER SEEDS	SESAME SEEDS
Phosphorus	2	4	1	3
Zinc	4	1	3	2
Magnesium	1	3	4	2
Vitamin E	2	4	1	3
Fiber	1	2	4	3
Omega-3	1	3	4	2
Polyunsaturated fat	2	4	1	3
Monounsaturated fat	3	4	2	1
Iron	2	4	3	1
Vitamin B6	3	4	1	2
Selenium	4	1	2	3
Saturated fat	3	4	1	2
Omega-6	3	2	4	1
Vitamin B1	1	4	3	2
Calcium	2	4	3	1
Vitamin C	2	3	1	4
1 = highest amount – 4 = lowest amount				

Source: USDA Food Composition Database

BLAME IT ON THE PHASE

Have you ever realized halfway through a jumbo bag of M&M's that you weren't even hungry in the first place? Don't worry ladies, I'm guilty as charged too. "My hormones made me do it" is a very common phrase I hear at my nutrition practice. Pesky hormones spewing from our brains and ovaries are to blame for magically transporting us from the couch to the kitchen and into that bag of salty potato chips or buttery popcorn. Gee, thanks hormones!

When it comes to our food choices, some may argue that these decisions are more or less out of our hands. Hormones are controlling our actions, our cravings, and even our desire (or lack of desire) to go back for seconds. Hormones can manipulate weight by shutting down hunger signals if we need to lose weight or rev up our appetite if we have to put on a few pounds. That being said, hormones don't just charge up our menstrual cycle, they dictate much more.

Curious to learn more? I thought so...

MAY I HAVE SECONDS OR THIRDS, PLEASE?

Physiologically, the body requires more energy from nutrients in the luteal phase (days 15 to 28), to continue building a fully developed uterine lining. The proof is in the pudding. Research found that women ate 685 calories/day more in the luteal phase than in the follicular and ovulatory phase.[37]

Thanks to the avalanche of hormones during the luteal phase, it's no wonder we feel more ravenous. Concentrations of progesterone are 12 to 20 times greater and estrogen concentration is three to four times higher in the luteal phase of the cycle compared to the follicular phase. Talk about a big spike in hormones!

Plus, according to research, we burn more calories (aka expend more energy) during the luteal phase, which prompts us to eat more.[38] If we are burning more calories, our body wants to fight that imbalance by pushing us closer and closer to the cookie jar. Additionally, there's an uptick in our metabolism (even when we sleep), causing us to feel a bit more inclined to have an extra snack or two, or three or four.

THE LUTEAL PHASE BRAIN WANTS WHAT IT WANTS: CARBS + FAT

The craving for carbs and fat is triggered by hormones in your brain, not just from your taste buds. In fact, numerous studies have found

37   https://www.sciencedirect.com/science/article/abs/pii/0031938494902968
38   https://www.ncbi.nlm.nih.gov/pubmed/1550036

that women eat more food, specifically carbohydrates and fats, in the luteal phase compared to the follicular phase. Here's why:

CARBOHYDRATES: Daydreaming about carbs is likely due to the fact that there's a plunge of mood-boosting serotonin around the same time that PMS strikes. When serotonin levels plummet, that drop adversely affects mood, prompts fatigue, and very noticeably heightens cravings. Carbs can easily bump serotonin levels back up because carbs increase the amino acid tryptophan, an important ingredient needed to make serotonin. That being said, don't knock yourself down if you succumb to tempting sweets and chocolates during this phase (especially for those with PMS). We are only human!

FATS: For all the butter and ice cream lovers, this one's for you. Basically, fatty acids are stolen from the brain to help rebuild the uterine lining (rude, I know). The brain mistakes this so-called robbery for having a shortage of fat in the bod. Therefore, our desire for fat-rich foods becomes amplified. Couple our infatuation for fat with spikes in the stress hormone cortisol right before our period and it's no wonder we want to curl up to a bowl of rich and velvety ice cream during the luteal phase. You had me at ice cream, say no more!

BUH-BYE HUNGER, HELLO HANKY-PANKY

As covered briefly during Food Cycling in Chapter 2, you may be less focused on eating when ovulation strikes. You may think "How rude?!," as Michelle Tanner from *Full House* puts it, but this predetermined biological decision comes along with a greater purpose. That's because during ovulation, testosterone (a hormone that boosts sexual desire) is high, estrogen (a natural appetite suppressant) is high, and ghrelin (a hunger hormone) is low. Thanks to these hormonal effects, we pay more attention to procreating and intercourse than to food. The shift in desire from food to fornicating is what has kept our breeding species alive, so please don't try to fight nature. Mmmokay!?

LOSING WEIGHT IN THE LUTEAL PHASE, NO WAY, JOSÉ!

Losing weight during the luteal phase is as unlikely as Jennifer Aniston and Brad Pitt getting back together. If the scale hasn't budged though you've been desperately trying to lose weight, it's not you, it's the hormones!

Why? Well, members of team progesterone are busy rebuilding the uterine lining. In fact, the upcoming period is relying on progesterone to get the job done and prepare the body for day 1 of the cycle. Therefore, we tend to eat more food to ensure that progesterone is well fed (and in good enough supply) in order to keep up with the physiological demands of the menstrual cycle. Although you expend more energy during sleep in the luteal phase than in the follicular phase and can burn more calories during the luteal phase when compared to the ovulatory phase, it is not an easy recipe for weight loss due to fluctuating hormones and stronger cravings.[39, 40] By default, weight loss can be very challenging during this phase.

39   https://www.ncbi.nlm.nih.gov/pubmed/3766447
40   https://www.ncbi.nlm.nih.gov/pubmed/2706224

A study in the *American Journal of Clinical Nutrition* tried to adapt a weight-loss program to healthy, overweight, premenopausal women by targeting changes in hunger hormones and cravings throughout the cycle. Interestingly enough, those who followed a diet tailored to counteract food cravings and hormones were able to lose an average of 9 pounds more than those who followed a standard diet. A strategy they used was to eat more protein and calories from healthy fats, such as nuts, seeds, and avocados during the luteal phase. And eating *some* dark chocolate instead of *all* the dark chocolate during the late luteal phase (when PMS strikes) was even allowed.[41] Rather than set yourself up for failure, you can work with the fluctuations of the menstrual cycle rather than compete against it. So, weight loss isn't necessarily impossible, but learning to work with the (hormone) cards you've been dealt is the key to success!

ONCE YOU POP, THE FUN DON'T STOP

If you've ever needed to be physically removed from the kitchen during the latter end of your cycle, you can blame those rambunctious hormones of yours! Around days 20 to 25 when both estrogen and progesterone are at their highest, binge eating and emotional eating are more likely to occur.[42, 43] Chronic dieters and those with disordered eating also have an increased risk for emotional eating and heightened cravings during this time. This makes physiological sense because we don't experience

41   https://academic.oup.com/ajcn/article/104/1/15/4569669
42   https://onlinelibrary.wiley.com/doi/full/10.1002/eat.22084
43   https://www.ncbi.nlm.nih.gov/pubmed/22889242

as much emotional eating during the first half of the cycle when progesterone isn't at bat yet.[44] Gee, thanks, progesterone!

Remember not to get frustrated at yourself if it does happen. I've put together helpful tools and strategies to stand up to those powerful hormones rather than having them knock you down. Just dust yourself off, you got this!

THE LUTEAL PHASE FOOD SOLUTIONS

CONTROL CARBOHYDRATE CRAVINGS: Don't lose hope entirely, we still have some control over what we eat! Give yourself carbohydrates during this phase and make sure to fill up on nutritious carbs such as brown rice, beans, fruit, and delicious and interesting whole grains like barley, farro, and wheat berries.

CONTROL SWEET CRAVINGS: Instead of going for refined or bleached sugars in cookies and muffins, have sources of sweets like antioxidant-rich dark chocolate, nut and seed butters, smoothies, and fresh or dried fruits such as dates, apricots, figs, or raisins. Although dried fruits may be high in natural sugar, you'll only need a few bites to satisfy your sweet tooth. Plus, dried fruit is high in potassium, which can tell your stress hormones to calm the hell down! Natural sugars are *sweet* indeed!

CONTROL FAT CRAVINGS: Foods rich in healthy monounsaturated and polyunsaturated fats, such as macadamia nuts, avocados, walnuts, and pumpkin seeds, are key to satisfying your body's

---

44   https://www.ncbi.nlm.nih.gov/pubmed/8623004

desire for fat. And foods with fat will show your sugar cravings who's boss by reducing your desire for sweet temptations.

CONTROL MAJOR HUNGER AND BOTTOMLESS PIT SYNDROME:

- Load your plate with non-starchy veggies, like tomatoes, celery, and bell peppers, to stay fuller longer, and eat more protein and fiber-rich foods to keep hunger at bay.

- Whatever you do, don't deny yourself the foods you want. By "allowing" yourself some carbs and sweets from the start, you'll be less likely to sneak them in and binge. It will lessen their allure and will stop you from putting these foods on a pedestal.

- Eat small, frequent meals instead of three big meals. This will allow you to look forward to your next meal, spread out your meal times, reduce insulin spikes, and give you more opportunities to satisfy your salt and sweet cravings with more food choices.

- Drink plenty of water to decrease potential bloating and to stay as regular as you can be.

BOOST SEROTONIN: Foods that help promote serotonin production, like brown rice, oats, and beans, should be emphasized in your diet. Remember that tryptophan plays a big role in serotonin production, so surround yourself with foods like spinach, salmon, and seeds to help turn that frown upside down.

REDUCE CORTISOL: Foods to fend off that stress hormone monster, cortisol, include antioxidant-rich foods such as blueberries, spinach, sweet potato, squash, and pomegranates. Plus, the vibrant pop in color from these nutritional gems may put a smile on your face, which automatically puts you in a better mood.

CONTROL CRAVINGS, NO MATTER THE PHASE:

- Acknowledge, accept, and plan for cravings so you can have food easily accessible when the cravings strike! Keep your pantry filled with whole grain crackers, nuts and seeds, dried fruit, and popcorn. If you fail to prepare, you may prepare to fail!

- Stock your fridge with precut or prewashed veggies like bell peppers, snap peas, or cucumber. That way you can nibble on those low-calorie, high-nutrient foods while deciding what to whip up for dinner.

- Eat more protein during your meals, such as eggs, beans, lentils, or bean-based pasta, to help you stay fuller for longer periods of time.

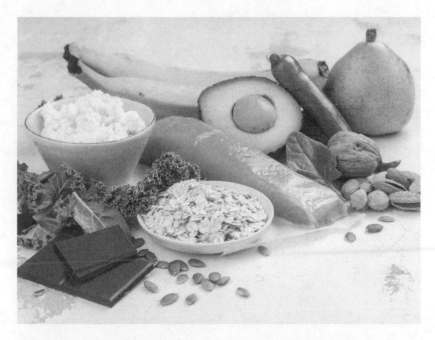

- Keep snacks in your purse and in your desk. There's no need to hit up the vending machine or go to the convenience store every time a craving hits. Buy a few different snacks you like in bulk and have them readily available in your purse or desk. You may also save money this way!

- Be careful with alcohol intake. Cravings for alcohol may go up as estrogen climbs starting around day 12. Give yourself a limit from the beginning of the night so you aren't peer-pressured to drink more. Sip your drink slowly, alternate between water and alcohol, and don't impulsively order another round of daiquiris if it wasn't your plan from the start.

- Chocolate is your friend! Dark chocolate (85% or higher cacao) can actually help calm you down thanks to the relaxing powers of magnesium.

- Don't get mad at yourself for having exorcism-like cravings some days. Keep calm and carry on!

5

PREMENSTRUAL DISORDERS

I once had a client coin herself as the Tasmanian devil the week leading up to her period. She was constantly in a frenzy, bloated AF, yelling at her husband, belittling her coworkers, and crying if someone dared to look at her the wrong way. All of a sudden her font went from normal to bold to italicized and underlined—all at the same time!

Welcome to the world of premenstrual syndrome (PMS). Feeling irritable, hangry, and super tired are common hormonal, physical, and emotional waves that millions of women experience in the days before their periods (and some experience PMS in the early days of their period!). But remember this: YOU ARE NOT ALONE. I encourage you to start to listen to your body ASAP because these symptoms are not normal my friends! Don't fret, because better nutrition can help you get through the challenges of PMS, so let's get started.

NOBODY PUTS THE HORMONES IN THE CORNER

I have good news and bad news. The bad news is that researchers have yet to land on a simple explanation of what causes PMS and PMDD (see A Closer Look at PMDD on page 73). But the good news is that we are *pretty* certain neurotransmitters and hormones are to blame. Sex hormones, like progesterone, testosterone, and estrogen, typically coexist throughout the entire menstrual cycle. But if one hormone decides to flex its muscle (*what a show-off*), it can throw the whole menstrual cycle off balance. Some women are extra sensitive to hormonal fluctuations while others are not, and those are just the facts of life. Plus, nutritional gaps in our diets can also claim responsibility as to why we experience PMS.

Other common potential causes include:

- Genetics[45]
- Change in hormone ratios
- Thyroid dysfunction
- Vitamin or mineral deficiency
- Essential fatty acid deficiency
- Decreased brain hormones, such as dopamine and serotonin.[46]

HOW DO I KNOW IF I HAVE IT?

PMS is one of the most common disorders in women. Roughly one in three women of reproductive age have one or more physical or

45   https://www.ajog.org/article/S0002-9378(17)30674-9/pdf
46   https://www.ncbi.nlm.nih.gov/pubmed/25363099

psychiatric symptoms related to PMS in the days leading up to their period.

Although there isn't a formal test, PMS is typically diagnosed if a woman reports at least one of the following symptoms (affective and somatic) during the five days before her period in at least three consecutive menstrual cycles.[47]

- *Affective symptoms:* Angry outbursts, anxiety, confusion, depression, irritability, social withdrawal
- *Somatic symptoms:* Abdominal bloating, breast tenderness or swelling, headache, joint or muscle pain, swelling of the extremities, weight gain

A CLOSER LOOK AT PMDD

PMS is on the lighter scale of intensity while premenstrual dysphoric disorder (PMDD) is classified as a severe, psychiatric, medical syndrome with clinical symptoms similar to those of depression. Those formally diagnosed with PMDD are often treated with medication and are routinely seen by a mental health professional. Affecting between 3% to 8% of women, PMDD deeply impacts a woman's life and can ruin relationships, tear families apart, and turn lives upside down.[48]

Although not an official test, the American Psychiatric Association developed criteria to help diagnose women with PMDD. Those with PMDD have at least 5 of the 11 following symptoms during the week before menses in at least two consecutive menstrual cycles. The

---

47 https://www.aafp.org/afp/2016/0801/p236.html
48 https://www.ajog.org/article/S0002-9378(17)30674-9/pdf

symptoms resolve within the first few days of their period.[49] These symptoms include:

- mood changes
- irritability/anger
- depression or hopelessness
- anxiety
- lack of interest in people/activities you enjoy
- difficulty concentrating
- fatigue or lack of energy
- appetite changes
- excessive sleepiness
- feeling overwhelmed
- physical symptoms (bloated, breast soreness or muscle pain)

For both PMS/PMDD, it's crucial to track symptoms in an app or in a symptom diary for a few months to help your gynecologist and/ or endocrinologist understand the timing, changes, duration, and severity of your ailments. This will also help health care providers distinguish symptoms from depression and anxiety, as PMDD/PMS are not present every day and can worsen cyclically. Sorry ladies, treatment isn't black and white so the more information you can collect, the better!

PMS SYMPTOMS

The timing of PMS symptoms is synonymous with being anxious before an exam. For instance, the week before the exam you are

---

49   Ibid.

really nervous, the day of the exam your nerves are spiraling out of control, but after the exam, you are cool as a cucumber. You may even act as if there was never an exam in the first place, *sheesh!* The days when you feel the most anxious are typically in line with when PMS symptoms are strongest.[50]

PMS symptoms are truly a mixed bag. The severity and cluster of symptoms differ from woman to woman. Just because your best girlfriend doesn't have the same breast pain or bloating you have doesn't mean that she doesn't have PMS.

Learn It, Live It, Love It

Don't be shamed or duped into thinking that PMS/PMDD is *just part of our journey as women,* and we have to roll up our sleeves and gear up every month for this roller-coaster ride. Don't brush symptoms under the rug and normalize them based on what society thinks. Stand up for your body, even if it means speaking openly and honestly about how you feel. A fantastic online community known as Period Space (http://periodspace.org or @hiperiodspace on Instagram) is designed to encourage public discussion on menstruation and destigmatize periods. It's been an incredible platform to lean on and a safe space to learn more.

Although general symptoms like bloating, sadness, and mood swings are common, these ailments can point the finger to an

---

50   https://www.ajog.org/article/S0002-9378(17)30674-9/pdf

underlying problem. Because the body does an incredible job of self-regulating and maintaining homeostasis, when we experience powerful emotional and physical symptoms, it means that something is internally off-kilter. Getting to the root of the problem by upping your nutrition game can help you say goodbye to PMS forever.

LET'S TREAT IT PLEASE!

When PMS hits, we are more drawn to want #foodporn (e.g., cheesy pasta, sweet and salty ice cream swirls, and gooey chocolate chip cookies). We find ourselves cozying up to treats to get out of the PMS "blech" funk. Sorry to break it to you but these quick fixes aren't the answer. In fact, they can make symptoms worse. Don't worry, better nutrition can help ward off unpleasant PMS symptoms. Specific nutrients, vitamins, and minerals are proven and recommended for PMS treatment because they simply know how to do the job, are cost-effective, are easily accessible, and happen to be delicious too.

In addition to eating more astutely, I advise clients to create a PMS symptom diary to record behaviors and out-of-the-blue characteristics for a handful of months. This will allow them to draw patterns from their recorded descriptions of moods, emotions, or physical symptoms—so I suggest you do the same! Keep it easy by using an app on your smartphone to track your symptoms. Be your own detective!

For some, medications and surgery may be warranted if symptoms and underlying medical pathologies become too severe. These women are advised to seek further medical attention and care from a multidisciplinary team such as a general practitioner, gynecologist, endocrinologist, mental health professional, and a registered dietitian. Please note that PMDD is a serious mental illness and requires more attention outside of nutritional guidance.

GENERAL PMS/PMDD GUIDELINES

These are the top ways to stand up to these imbalances through better nutrition, stat!

1. Eat small, frequent meals throughout the day to curb cravings and stabilize blood sugar.

2. Get ahead of snack cravings and arm yourself with real nutrition coming from easy snacks like fruit, yogurt, nuts, cheese, or popcorn.

3. Focus on feel-good foods from omega-3s, such as salmon, olive oil, and walnuts to boost mood and ward off mood swings by keeping blood sugar balanced.

4. Eat at least one square of dark chocolate per day to help boost mood and lessen anxiety.

5. Reduce high amounts of fruit juice, soda, and alcohol, as they can worsen PMS. If there isn't any fiber to slow down the rapid absorption of carbohydrates, it will send your blood sugar on a massive roller-coaster ride.

6. Eat wholesome, antioxidant-filled carbs like sweet potato, butternut squash, and parsnips.

7. Avoid PMS constipation and eat fiber-rich foods (oats, pears, berries, whole grains) to promote regularity and keep you feeling fuller longer, especially when hunger kicks in more frequently.

8. Avoid PMS diarrhea and eat more anti-inflammatory foods with omega-3 fatty acids, like salmon and flaxseeds, or colorful fruits and vegetables, like berries, zucchini, and sweet potatoes.

9. To keep your gut health in check, eat probiotic-rich food like yogurt or kefir, prebiotic-rich foods like oats, bananas, and garlic, or consider a probiotic with *Lactobacillus* or *Bifidobacterium*.

10. Drink water or herbal teas to decrease water retention and bloating.

11. Take a well-balanced multivitamin every day. See each section for more specifics but generally:

- Vitamin D3, cholecalciferol, 400 to 800IU
- Magnesium, magnesium citrate, 200 to 400mg
- Vitamin B6, 100mg
- Vitamin B1, 1.1mg
- Vitamin E, 400IU
- Calcium, calcium carbonate, 1,000 to 1,200mg/day or 500 to 600mg 2x/day
- DHA/EPA omega-3s, 1,500 to 2,000mg

NOTE: If you have severe PMS/PMDD/dysmenorrhea, talk to your MD about taking an additional 50 to 100mg/day a day of vitamin B6, not exceeding 200mg/day to prevent nerve damage and liver toxicity.

CAUTION: The Food and Drug Administration (FDA) does not regulate any vitamin or mineral and herbal supplements the way they regulate medications, so talk to your doctor before taking any supplements. They may interact with other medications you take and may cause dangerous effects.

NUTRIENTS TO BE RECKONED WITH

Food is not the enemy in PMS, it is actually your bestie. Like I said before, menstruation in and of itself is an inflammatory process, which is why we want to eat foods to keep inflammation at bay, keep hormones balanced and reduce maddening menstrual cramps. Think of all of the following nutrients as the powerful and dynamic girls that make up your sorority. Individually, they are fierce members of the group, helping to make *ish* happen on campus. Some of them are leaders, while others make sure everything is going smoothly from the sidelines or behind the scenes. But as a group, they are a force to be reckoned with because together, nobody, not even PMS or your arch rival sorority, can stand in your way. Meet your chapter members ladies:

VITAMIN B6, PYRIDOXINE

Without enough vitamin B6, say goodbye to serotonin. Trust me, during PMS, you want a lot of this mood-boosting brain chemical. Lots of research has found that vitamin B6 can manage moodiness, irritability, bloating, and anxiety associated with PMS.

WHAT THE RESEARCH SAYS

- Doses of 100mg/day of vitamin B6 significantly improves overall PMS symptoms such as depression, irritability, and tiredness.[51, 52]

TRACY'S TAKEAWAYS

1. Take 100mg of vitamin B6 daily. It is not recommended to go above 200mg/day in supplement form because toxic effects have been found in research.

2. Eat vitamin B6-rich foods such as turkey, lentils, fish, potatoes, non-citrus fruits like banana and watermelon, poultry, and fortified cereals.

VITAMIN B1, THIAMINE

This water-soluble vitamin can basically bring you back to life when PMS is in town. Thiamine breaks down carbs so more mood-boosting neurotransmitters are available in the brain (such as serotonin and dopamine). Thiamine can also improve circulation to dissolve cramps when PMS strikes. Thanks to thiamine, say peace out to gloomy clouds, and say hello to beautiful blue skies.

WHAT THE RESEARCH SAYS

- Thiamine has helped reduce both mental and physical pain symptoms of PMS. It has been shown to boost endorphin secretion, which expands blood vessels, helping to relieve PMS pain.[53]

51   https://www.ncbi.nlm.nih.gov/pmc/articles/PMC27878/
52   https://www.ajog.org/article/S0002-9378(17)30674-9/pdf
53   https://www.ncbi.nlm.nih.gov/pubmed/25363099

- Over a period of 10 years, women with higher dietary intakes of thiamine had a significantly lower risk of PMS.[54, 55]

TRACY'S TAKEAWAYS

1. Aim for 1.1mg per day of thiamine in your multivitamin.

2. Enjoy thiamine-rich foods, including oats, whole grain or bean-based pasta, nuts, oranges, rice, sesame seeds, and flaxseeds.

OMEGA-3 FATTY ACIDS

PMS won't even stand a chance against the mighty anti-inflammatory effects of omega-3s. Two main forms of omega-3 fatty acids, eicosapentaenoic acid (EPA) and docosahexaenoic acid (DHA), act as inflammation and pain squashers that your body craves and truly appreciates during PMS. Why? Well...

Cramp-contributing omega-6 lipid compounds known as prostaglandins (that have been busy rebuilding the uterine lining since ovulation) finally reach their peak during PMS. Right before your period, prostaglandins stimulate muscles that break down and release the uterine lining, causing your uterus to feel like it's pulsing like an Avicii techno beat and your breasts to feel hard as a rock. *Lovely, I know.*

In general, the more pulsating, proinflammatory prostaglandins in the uterus (side note: this *could* be a sign of endometriosis), the more likely you are to have pain, tenderness, and distention. However, the anti-inflammatory properties of omega-3s can put the kibosh on the prostaglandins responsible for pain. Yahoo! To conclude, more omega-3 foods = fewer cramps.

---

54 https://www.ncbi.nlm.nih.gov/pubmed/2558186
55 https://www.ncbi.nlm.nih.gov/pubmed/23444100

WHAT THE RESEARCH SAYS

- Taking omega-3s for 45 days reduced anxiety, low concentration, bloating, and depression more than a placebo. After 90 days, in addition to those symptoms, nervousness, headache, and breast tenderness all decreased.[56]

- Omega-3s could be an acceptable form of treatment in mild cases of depression and for painful periods.[57]

TRACY'S TAKEAWAYS

1. Take 1500 to 2000mg of DHA/EPA omega-3s to improve PMS symptoms.

2. The standard American diet is low in omega-3, so stock up on sources like flaxseeds, almonds, walnuts, omega-3 fortified eggs, pumpkin seeds, and salmon. Because you may be wanting more food during this phase, have more protein coming from omega-3s to keep you fuller longer.

VITAMIN D

Vitamin D plays a critical role in reproductive health and mood regulation, and has been a hot-button topic in its relationship to PMS. During PMS, estrogen dips suddenly, causing us to feel anything but perfect. Plummeting estrogen also takes down vitamin D, hinting at a close-knit relationship between these two lovebirds– watch out Bradley Cooper and Lady Gaga! See page 25 in Food Cycling for more about vitamin D.

---

56   https://www.ncbi.nlm.nih.gov/pubmed/23642943
57   https://www.ncbi.nlm.nih.gov/pubmed/12642146

Seasonal Affective Disorder

Seasonal affective disorder (SAD) is linked to low vitamin D from lack of sunlight, especially in high-latitude countries, so it's no wonder you aren't filled with mood-boosting serotonin during those dreary, darker winter months. Brain hormones such as serotonin and dopamine are activated by vitamin D, so in the colder and darker months, you may not be your peppy self. In a research study, Canadians were found to be low in vitamin D because of less winter sun exposure, which in turn increased their risk for PMS.[58]

WHAT THE RESEARCH SAYS

- When compared to those with high vitamin D, those with low vitamin D were more likely to have cramps, fatigue, anxiety, and low libido in the days leading up to their periods.[59]

- Vitamin D supplements improve PMS-related mood symptoms, such as depression and anxiety. [60, 61]

- High doses of vitamin D supplements (one 50,000IU dose per week under medical supervision) over the course of nine weeks decreased the prevalence of PMS, backache, tendency to cry, and painful periods.[62]

- Over 10 years, a diet high in vitamin D reduced the development of PMS when compared to a diet low in vitamin D.[63]

58   https://www.ncbi.nlm.nih.gov/pubmed/30177298
59   https://www.ncbi.nlm.nih.gov/pubmed/30177298
60   https://www.ncbi.nlm.nih.gov/pubmed/26724745
61   https://www.ncbi.nlm.nih.gov/pmc/articles/PMC4815371/
62   https://www.ncbi.nlm.nih.gov/pubmed/29447494
63   https://www.ncbi.nlm.nih.gov/pubmed/15956003

TRACY'S TAKEAWAYS

1. Aim for 400 to 800IU of vitamin D/day. Look for the active form, vitamin D3, cholecalciferol on the bottle.

2. Load up on vitamin D-rich foods such as milk, orange juice, fatty fish (salmon, mackerel, tuna), egg yolk, cheese, mushrooms, and breakfast cereals. Research found that women who ate a diet high in vitamin D reduced their risk of PMS by 40%.[64]

CALCIUM

Calcium, the mineral we associate with our teeth and bones, may have a role in relieving anxiety, a common symptom of PMS. When PMS is in town, anxiety is usually cranked up in the brain and calcium-rich foods may hold the power to turn down the anxiety volume. Low calcium is also thought to be a big contributor to PMS. In fact, researchers strongly believe that PMS may actually be a sign of calcium deficiency. In PMS, just like how vitamin D declines when estrogen starts to plummet, calcium also scurries away and goes MIA. *Gasp!* After reading this, is anyone else craving some calcium-rich cheese? I'll meet you in the kitchen!

WHAT THE RESEARCH SAYS

- Taking 500mg of calcium showed significant positive differences in anxiety, depression, and bloating after the first mentrual cycle and even more positive differences were noticed after the second menstrual cycle.[65] PMS-related depression and sadness were significantly more reduced in women who received calcium supplementation than those who received a placebo.[66]

---

64   Ibid.
65   https://www.ncbi.nlm.nih.gov/pubmed/28217679
66   https://www.ncbi.nlm.nih.gov/pubmed/19574172

- Calcium treatment of 1200mg/day after three months resulted in an approximate 50% reduction in symptoms such as depression, mood swings, headache, and irritability. Calcium also decreased moodiness, water retention such as bloating, food cravings, and period pain.[67]

- Bloating was significantly reduced with calcium supplementation of 1200mg/day or eating 1200mg of calcium per day.[68, 69]

- When compared to women who eat a lower intake of calcium (528mg/day), those with higher calcium intake from food sources (1283mg/day) had a lower risk of developing PMS.[70] Fifty-five percent of women experienced relief from PMDD symptoms after taking calcium carbonate supplements for three months.[71]

Vitamin D + Calcium Connection

In the US, many women do not eat the recommended amount of calcium and vitamin D per day. Did you know that calcium is essentially powerless without vitamin D? Vitamin D basically provides the wheels so calcium can cruise along the digestive tract and then distribute itself to the places where the body needs calcium the most, like the bones and kidneys. Otherwise, calcium would uselessly slide in and out of the body in the blink of an eye. So, bump up both your calcium and vitamin D intake, stat! Your body is desperate for it!

67   https://www.ncbi.nlm.nih.gov/pubmed/9731851
68   Ibid.
69   https://www.ncbi.nlm.nih.gov/pubmed/8498421
70   https://www.ncbi.nlm.nih.gov/pubmed/15956003
71   https://www.ncbi.nlm.nih.gov/pubmed/9731851

TRACY'S TAKEAWAYS

1. Take 1,000 to 1,200mg calcium carbonate for at least three months to help improve PMS symptoms.

2. Calcium is a MUST. Calcium-rich foods include salmon, bok choy, kale, white beans, tofu, and almonds. However, if you have a history of kidney stones, please talk to your doctor before supplementing with calcium as it may make you more prone to kidney stone development.

3. Have dairy! Skim or low-fat milk is associated with a lower risk of PMS.[72]

MAGNESIUM

Magnesium to the rescue!

Magnesium can help to relax muscle contractions coming from the uterus during PMS. Progesterone (a natural muscle relaxer) declines during the last few days of the luteal phase so it's typical to have more pelvic pain creeping up. That being said, it's super important to eat enough magnesium to decrease cramping but also to improve sleep quality, lower stress levels, build more serotonin levels, and even aid in the production of progesterone. Plus, magnesium may be helpful for menstrual migraines often associated with PMS.

So, if you are feeling particularly irritable and not so easy to please, it's possible that PMS is really masking a magnesium deficiency or insufficiency. Similar to calcium and vitamin D, women with PMS also appear to have low levels of magnesium, *shreek!* Now that's something to think about!

---

72   https://www.ncbi.nlm.nih.gov/pubmed/15956003

Three Helpful Nutrients

Calcium, magnesium, and vitamin D were found to be low in women with PMS so make sure your meals are rounded with this trio. Plus, this combo is helpful in the relief of constipation.[73] Have:

Greek yogurt + pumpkin seeds + blackberries

Whole grain breakfast cereal + slivered almonds + soy milk

Or salmon + mushrooms + broccoli

WHAT THE RESEARCH SAYS

- Magnesium supplementation has been shown to relieve PMS symptoms and may help to relieve bloating and improve mood.[74]

- Supplementing with 200mg of magnesium plus 50mg of vitamin B6 for one month can reduce anxiety, nervous tension, mood swings, and irritability related to PMS.[75] Vitamin B6 may increase the absorption of magnesium, which is why these two supplements work well in harmony.

- Magnesium deficiency may result in thyroid conditions (such as secondary hyperparathyroidism or hypoparathyroidism) manifesting as symptoms similar to PMS.[76]

TRACY'S TAKEAWAYS

1. Aim for 200 to 400mg of magnesium citrate to help reduce bloating. It may also help you go to the bathroom if you are experiencing

73   https://www.ncbi.nlm.nih.gov/pmc/articles/PMC4667262
74   https://www.ncbi.nlm.nih.gov/pubmed/2067759
75   https://www.ncbi.nlm.nih.gov/pubmed/10746516
76   https://www.ncbi.nlm.nih.gov/pubmed/9731851

PMS-related constipation. Opt for magnesium glycinate for a more gentle effect if you have no issues going #2.

2. Consume magnesium-rich foods, including pumpkin seeds, brown rice, flaxseeds, chickpeas, peanuts, artichokes, sweet potato, and almonds.

SEROTONIN AND COMPLEX CARBOHYDRATES

It's not exactly a nutrient, but serotonin is a feel-good brain chemical worth discussing. Hormones continue to head south during PMS, leaving you with cravings, hunger pangs, and a smile turned upside down. That's because serotonin and estrogen, both responsible for regulating and balancing mood, are barely hanging by a thread during PMS so you aren't your cheery, energized self. Research has found that those with PMS overconsume carbohydrates as a placeholder for happiness with hopes of removing themselves from this slump.[77, 78] Understanding how the brain works during PMS has been instrumental because antidepressant medications, such as selective serotonin reuptake inhibitors (SSRIs), have been found to be an effective treatment for PMS.[79]

WHAT THE RESEARCH SAYS

- Intense carbohydrate cravings could be linked to low serotonin in the brain. A diet rich in complex carbohydrates during the luteal phase helped relieve PMS because carbohydrates boost serotonin production.[80]

---

77 https://www.ncbi.nlm.nih.gov/pmc/articles/PMC1327664/#B41
78 https://www.ncbi.nlm.nih.gov/pubmed/2589444
79 https://www.ajog.org/article/S0002-9378(17)30674-9/pdf
80 https://www.ncbi.nlm.nih.gov/pubmed/7675373

- Overeating maltose, a starch generally found in bagels, frozen desserts, hard candies, and processed cereals, can increase the risk for PMS.[81]

TRACY'S TAKEAWAYS

1. Add a variety of complex carbohydrates into your diet, such as farro, beans, brown rice, and quinoa.

2. Eat small, frequent meals instead of three large meals to help sprinkle mood-boosting serotonin throughout your day.

CHROMIUM

Chromium, a trace mineral, may play a role in blood sugar control, mood, and insulin production. While limited research has been done to the present date, due to its promising relationship in PMDD management, I have a feeling more research on its way.

WHAT THE RESEARCH SAYS

- A small study on women with PMDD with a poor quality of life showed that taking chromium supplements for one month reduced mood symptoms and improved overall health satisfaction.[82]

TRACY'S TAKEAWAYS

1. Get chromium through food sources such as whole grains, bran cereals, fruits like oranges and grapes, and veggies like potatoes and broccoli.

2. If you have PMDD, talk to your doctor about supplementing short term with chromium picolinate.

---

81   https://www.ncbi.nlm.nih.gov/pubmed/29379144
82   https://www.ncbi.nlm.nih.gov/pubmed/24237190

MANGANESE

Manganese levels fluctuate throughout the menstrual cycle, along with other essential nutrients like zinc, iron, and magnesium. Because of its strong association with mood swings associated with PMS, manganese may be a hot nutrient in research down the road.

WHAT THE RESEARCH SAYS

- Manganese can lead to fewer pain symptoms and better mood.[83]

TRACY'S TAKEAWAYS

Eat manganese-rich foods such as sweet potato, nuts, and wheat germ.

ARGININE

During PMS, arginine, an essential amino acid, can function as a shield against harmful stress and inflammation. Arginine is converted to nitric oxide in the blood, and we should learn to love nitric oxide. Nitric oxide expands our tiny and constricted blood vessels, which can increase helpful blood flow to the ovaries and uterus. Young adults with PMS have been shown to have elevated diastolic blood pressure (the top number in a blood pressure reading, so it would be "120" in a reading of 120/80), and arginine can help combat high blood pressure.[84]

WHAT THE RESEARCH SAYS

- Arginine may decrease inflammation in the uterus.[85]

---

83   https://www.ncbi.nlm.nih.gov/pubmed/8498421
84   https://www.ncbi.nlm.nih.gov/pmc/articles/PMC5116659/
85   https://www.ncbi.nlm.nih.gov/pubmed/21430253

- Animals receiving arginine treatments show less oxidative stress and higher-quality ovarian tissue during the luteal phase.[86]

TRACY'S TAKEAWAYS

Sprinkle some arginine-rich foods to your diet, including dark chocolate, pumpkin seeds, watermelon seeds, hemp seeds, and beets.

PROBIOTICS

Probiotics are having a moment, for all the right reasons. From drinks to supplements, everyone is trying to infuse their life with more gut-friendly probiotics.

Probiotics are beneficial strains of healthy bacteria and yeast that hang out in your digestive tract. Probiotics can help with a bevy of conditions such as improving immune function, regulating mood, reducing anxiety, healing the gut, and boosting brain power. If there is too much bad bacteria lurking, probiotics help build your army of good bacteria in the gut to correct this imbalance.

For example, when PMS strikes, we are more likely to experience some bathroom woes thanks to hormonal fluctuations. Probiotics can help keep your gut health in check, especially if you experience a surplus of gas, bloating, diarrhea, or even constipation related to PMS. To your surprise, the gut also helps to regulate hormones. Therefore, if the gut isn't working up to speed, hormonal imbalances can be the reason why some women experience PMS in the first place. So yes, it's possible that probiotics may help to ward off PMS.

---

86   https://www.ncbi.nlm.nih.gov/pubmed/29501008

WHAT THE RESEARCH SAYS

- Specific probiotic strains, *Bifidobacterium* and *Lactobacillus*, can improve psychiatric disorder-related behaviors such as anxiety, depression, and OCD.[87]

- The specific strain, *Lactobacillus rhamnosus*, has been found to show significant potential for reducing anxiety by releasing GABA, a neurotransmitter which can calm your brain.[88]

TRACY'S TAKEAWAYS

1. If you are looking to manage PMS-related anxiety, flourish your gut with probiotic superbugs coming from foods such as yogurt, quark, kefir, miso, apple cider vinegar, sauerkraut, kombucha, and kimchi.

2. To help reduce stress and anxiety, consider taking a supplement.

DISCLAIMER: We can't 100% say that all probiotic supplements hold up against strong acid during the digestive process; however, we can rely on food to make it through the digestive system unscathed.

ANTIOXIDANTS

Oxidative stress, stemming from lack of sleep, a poor diet, or even environmental pollutants, can potentially poke holes at otherwise perfect hormones, causing them to start to drag in the bod. In fact, research has shown that those with PMS were found to have low amounts of antioxidants (specifically glutathione), especially during the luteal phase.[89] Eating foods that are rich in antioxidants can repair damaged hormones and get them back up to speed in no time.

---

87   https://www.ncbi.nlm.nih.gov/pubmed/27413138
88   https://www.ncbi.nlm.nih.gov/pmc/articles/PMC6010276/
89   https://link.springer.com/article/10.1007%2Fs00404-009-1347-y

WHAT THE RESEARCH SAYS

- Vitamin E, a powerful antioxidant, has been shown to help lessen breast pain and tenderness associated with PMS.[90]

TRACY'S TAKEAWAYS

1. Take 400IU of vitamin E during the luteal phase to help prevent PMS and breast pain.

2. Selenium-rich foods contain glutathione, a powerful antioxidant, so aim for more Brazil nuts, sesame seeds, garlic, and shallots.

3. If cramps are out of control, it may be beneficial to swap to a more antioxidant-rich, plant-based diet for at least two months, which may reduce PMS symptoms and cramping.[91]

CAFFEINE

Let's cut to the chase. Caffeine was not associated with PMS in research, and women can still drink their coffee without fear that it will directly cause PMS.[92] However, let's be honest about what caffeine does to the body. It's a natural diuretic (meaning you urinate more), which can lead to bloat, abdominal discomfort, and bathroom troubles, all of which are very common symptoms in PMS. Plus, excess caffeine may block the exit pathway for estrogen, causing a buildup of estrogen in the bod. Although, there isn't a direct association between caffeine and PMS, a word to the wise would be to sip with caution, especially if your PMS just won't give.

---

90   https://journals.lww.com/greenjournal/Abstract/2003/05000/Clinical_Management_Guidelines_For.52.aspx
91   https://www.ncbi.nlm.nih.gov/pubmed/10674588
92   https://academic.oup.com/ajcn/article/104/2/499/4564558

WHAT THE RESEARCH SAYS

- Women who had 4 cups or more of coffee a day vs. those who did not drink coffee had a 68% increase in estradiol (the active form of estrogen) during their periods, which led to cramps, acne, and bloating.[93]

- Regardless of the caffeine sourced from tea, cola, coffee, or caffeinated soft drinks, women consuming 500mg of caffeine had a 71% increase in estradiol vs. those who had <100mg of caffeine per day.[94]

The Caffeine in Your Cup

1 cup hot coffee = ~160mg caffeine

1 ounce espresso = ~64mg caffeine

1 cup cold brew = ~100mg caffeine

1 cup green tea = ~40mg caffeine

1 cup black tea = ~50mg caffeine

1 cup cola = ~35mg

TRACY'S TAKEAWAYS

1. Aim for moderate intake. Why?... Well, no matter the source, caffeine can bump up the risk for stress, irritability, anxiety, rapid heart rate, high blood pressure, and impaired sleep quality. It's advised to moderate or eliminate caffeine intake to help curb these symptoms.

---

93   https://www.ncbi.nlm.nih.gov/pubmed/11591405
94   Ibid.

2. Rampant hormonal fluctuations and other menstrual discomfort during PMS may prevent you from getting some high-quality shut-eye. Coupling these woes with excessive caffeine may not be the ideal recipe for a good night's slumber.

3. PMS naturally puts you into snoozeville and caffeine can look extra-appealing when PMS strikes. Caffeine's jolt may be a quick fix but makes you more likely to depend on it rather fix the root of the issue (e.g., thumbing through Instagram feeds late at night, not having a proper wind-down routine, watching heart-racing shows before bedtime).

4. If caffeine naturally makes you more jittery and anxious, mixing caffeine with PMS symptoms can add fuel to the fire. Everyone's response to caffeine is different, so pay attention to your body. Monitor sleep quality, mood, and heart rate to help you land on the right amount. If you'd rather just NOT right now with caffeine, opt for herbal decaf teas, such as ginger or chamomile tea, infused water, kombuchas, seltzers, and decaffeinated beverages.

ALCOHOL

Alcohol is another hot-button topic when it comes to PMS development and management. Several studies have shown that PMS tends to be more severe among women who drink alcohol. It isn't 100% clear whether it can be blamed on the alcohol itself or whether PMS-prone women reach for the bottle more to better cope with their PMS-related symptoms. Regardless, alcohol can have disrupting effects on the body such as bloating, dehydration, heightened cravings and can exacerbate PMS-related symptoms.

WHAT THE RESEARCH SAYS

- A thorough systematic review and meta-analysis of studies involving more than 47,000 women concluded that alcohol intake presents a moderate association with PMS risk, increasing the risk to 45%, while heavy drinkers had a 79% heightened risk of PMS.[95]

- Alcohol may amplify PMS by altering levels of sex steroid hormones, proinflammatory markers, and gonadotropins like FSH and LH.

- Alcohol may interfere with the production of mood balancing chemicals in the brain, such as serotonin.

TRACY'S TAKEAWAYS

1. It may be wise to pull back on the alcohol front, especially if you have recurring PMS and breast tenderness. Pay attention to how alcohol makes you feel and modify accordingly.

2. Always opt for moderation when it comes to alcohol consumption.

TRACY'S PMS SYMPTOM MANAGEMENT

BLOATING: Reduce caffeine and alcohol, increase probiotics rich food, increase magnesium, increase calcium, increase omega-3

ANXIETY, NERVOUSNESS, AND MOOD SWINGS: Try *Lactobacillus rhamnosus*, increase magnesium, increase serotonin food boosters, increase complex carbohydrates, increase calcium, increase vitamin D,

---

95   https://www.ncbi.nlm.nih.gov/pubmed/29661913

increase manganese, increase omega-3, increase vitamin B6, increase vitamin B1

BELLY ISSUES: Reduce caffeine and alcohol, increase probiotic rich food, increase calcium

HEADACHE: Reduce caffeine and alcohol, increase calcium, increase omega-3

CRAVINGS: Reduce alcohol, increase calcium, increase complex carbohydrates

PAIN OR CRAMPS: Reduce caffeine and alcohol, increase serotonin food boosters, increase calcium, increase vitamin D, omega-3, increase complex carbohydrates, increase vitamin B1

FATIGUE OR INSOMNIA: Reduce caffeine and alcohol, increase calcium, increase vitamin D, increase complex carbohydrates, increase vitamin B6

BREAST TENDERNESS: Increase vitamin E, reduce alcohol, increase antioxidants, increase calcium, increase omega-3

PMDD: Increase calcium, increase chromium

GENERAL PMS: Reduce caffeine and alcohol; increase antioxidants, increase probiotic-rich food, increase arginine-rich food, increase serotonin food boosters, increase calcium, increase vitamin D, increase omega-3, increase vitamin B6, increase vitamin B1. See resources (page 264) for more forms of PMS treatments.

OTHER IMPORTANT TREATMENTS: Keep a symptom diary, set boundaries, prioritize what is essential, slow down, and rest often!

6

POLYCYSTIC OVARIAN SYNDROME

It's not easy being perfect all the time! We can't expect our hair to look fresh and full, our skin to look bright and flawless, and to be in a peppy, optimistic mood constantly. As much as we strive every day to look and feel our absolute best, for some of us, it can be nearly impossible. Why? Blame it on hormonal imbalances. They are preventing a lot of us from living our best life.

At my nutrition practice, the most common hormonal conditions that I've worked with include:

- Polycystic ovarian syndrome (PCOS)
- Endometriosis
- Thyroid dysfunction (Hashimoto's disease, hypothyroidism, and hyperthyroidism)
- Amenorrhea
- Infertility

Of course, there is a laundry list of other hormonal and reproductive conditions that can offset your period, your mood and energy, and your libido, but in this and the chapters that follow, I'm going to focus on what you can do about the above diagnoses with a FOOD FIRST approach.

WHAT IS PCOS?

PCOS is a common disorder of the endocrine system that I see so often at my practice. It's a complex, hormonal imbalance that affects the whole entire body, from the reproductive system to the endocrine and nervous systems.

Health risks associated with PCOS include high blood pressure, cardiovascular disease, diabetes, inflammation, weight gain, difficulty losing weight, heightened food cravings, high cholesterol, mood disorders (anxiety and depression), and increased risk for reproductive cancers such as breast, endometrial, uterine, and ovarian. High amounts of androgens (aka male hormones) is a characteristic of PCOS that leads to symptoms such as acne, hirsutism (hair growth in male places such as chin, sideburns, and chest), male pattern hair loss (horseshoe baldness), and difficulty losing weight. PCOS can present itself in obese, overweight, average, or underweight women. Regardless of weight, women can have symptoms such as insulin resistance or cysts on their ovaries.

PCOS is one of the leading causes of infertility in women because it causes a glitch in our reproductive system and can stop follicle development and ovulation. Women with PCOS may be at a higher risk to menstruate less often, and those with larger waist circumferences have been associated with more menstrual cycle disorders that negatively impact their fertility.[96]

HOW DO I KNOW IF I HAVE IT?

A common (but not universal) tool used to diagnose PCOS is using the Rotterdam Criteria, where two out of the following three criteria are needed to be diagnosed:[97]

1. **Ovulation dysfunction.** This can be either oligomenorrhea OR anovulation.

2. **Hyperandrogenism.** This is based on *clinical symptoms* (alopecia, acne, hirsutism, dark or excessive hair growth) OR *biochemical symptoms* (elevated testosterone, dihydrotestosterone, or androstenedione).

3. **Polycystic (small cysts) ovaries.** This is seen during an ultrasound.

Your doctor may be able to diagnose you but there is no definitive hallmark criteria for PCOS, and the diagnosis can often be subjective. A formal diagnosis can be made with ovarian biopsy but this is not a common practice. Elevated levels of insulin, luteinizing hormone (LH), and androgen hormones may be found in the blood during routine testing, but not all the time. This highlights the importance of being your own advocate by logging changes in mood and symptoms such as dark hair, weight changes, acne, or cycle irregularity. Bring all of this helpful information to your medical

96   https://www.ncbi.nlm.nih.gov/pubmed/29124856
97   https://bmcmedicine.biomedcentral.com/articles/10.1186/s12916-015-0299-2

professional's attention during routine checkups. Remember to ask questions and look for trends in lab values to extrapolate any major changes.

HOW DID I GET IT?

Unfortunately, there is no clear-cut answer for this one, gals. It's a lot of everything... it's the environment, lifestyle, inflammation, hormonal imbalances, as well as genetics. PCOS can also emerge in times of significant stress. But there is one major contributing factor in a large percentage of women with PCOS: insulin resistance.

After you eat, the pancreas releases the hormone insulin to balance the sugar in the blood. Insulin helps to fuel your body by soaking in nutrients and sugar from the blood and distributing it to hungry muscle, fat, and liver cells, which keeps your body moving and grooving.

However, 70% of women with PCOS have insulin resistance, which is when the body becomes "resistant" to insulin. The cells don't respond well to insulin anymore and the body will build up a tolerance to it. Though insulin is trying its best to get the body to take in nutrients, the body becomes stubborn and just doesn't want to listen. The cells, once energized by the valuable nutrients delivered by insulin, are now left high and dry. Sugar ends up sitting in the bloodstream, which can cause fatigue, brain fog, and massive carb cravings. In response, the body tells the pancreas to make more insulin (because it's hungry!), but the pancreas gets tired, and frankly annoyed, by this demanding request. Eventually, this increased workload leads to insulin resistance and potentially other serious health problems down the road, such as type 2 diabetes. The good news is that insulin resistance can be reversed through behavior, diet, and lifestyle changes.

MANAGEMENT OF PCOS

I have a lot of nutrition tips up my sleeve to help you better manage PCOS. Recognizing the symptoms early and being proactive will greatly reduce your long-term health risks. By improving insulin sensitivity through better-for-you food choices, your cells will become retrained in regulating insulin while damaged insulin will be escorted out of the building!

Treating PCOS is not a one-size-fits-all approach. Individualized treatment is really important, so work with a professional to tailor this advice more to your personal goals and needs. Remember, PCOS comes in all shapes and sizes so some of these approaches may not be for you, which is OK!

YOUR DIET

Women with PCOS who ate well and exercised regularly were able to get their hormones under control and manage insulin better.[98] A thorough Cochrane report showed that diet, exercise, and lifestyle modification was typically the first line of defense for overweight and obese women with PCOS. That being said, if you are overweight, it could positively improve your health to lose weight. Dropping 5% to 10% of your body weight may help to restore ovulation cycles, improve cycle regularity, improve insulin resistance, reduce high levels of androgens, improve fertility, and improve pregnancy rates for those going through fertility treatments.[99] In a study, 90% of

98   https://www.ncbi.nlm.nih.gov/pubmed?term=21328294
99   https://www.ncbi.nlm.nih.gov/pubmed/28416368

obese women who lost 20 pounds resumed ovulation and greatly increased their chances for pregnancy.[100] Reducing excess body fat may be the key to restoring reproductive, hormonal balance, insulin sensitivity, and metabolic functioning. I want to reiterate, not all women are insulin resistant and not all women have to lose weight, so it's important to follow a plan that works for YOU.

SO WHAT DIET WORKS BEST?

At this time, there is no clear and definitive evidence that one type of diet is superior to another in PCOS management. When appropriate and regardless of how it was achieved, weight loss has been shown to improve menstruation and reproduction without medical intervention or medication. However, don't decrease your calories too low or do anything dangerous in order to lose weight—a drop in food intake below 1,500 calories can drastically slow down metabolism and put a damper on sleep, digestion, mood, and concentration. Yikes!

Some researchers believe low-carb/low-glycemic index (GI) diets may lead to less insulin production, but that's not an across-the-board recommendation. A meta-analysis compared all types of diets for PCOS management. See Breaking Down the Diet on page 104. Overweight and obese women with PCOS who followed a low-carbohydrate, ketogenic diet (limiting their carbohydrate intake to 20 grams or less per day for 24 weeks) significantly reduced body weight by 12% and improved fasting insulin by 54%.[101] A study showed that a high-protein/low-carb diet (30% protein, 40% carbohydrates, 30% fat) and a low-protein/high-carb diet (15% protein, 55% carbohydrates, 30% fat) were both equally effective

---

100   https://www.ncbi.nlm.nih.gov/pubmed/9688382
101   https://www.ncbi.nlm.nih.gov/pmc/articles/PMC1334192

for weight loss and both diets improved insulin resistance, high cholesterol, and fat.[102]

Breaking Down the Diet for PCOS

PURPOSE	TYPE OF EATING PLAN
Weight loss	Monounsaturated fat-enriched diet
Improved menstrual regularity	Low-glycemic-index diet
Reduction in insulin and cholesterol	Low-carbohydrate, low-glycemic-index diet
Improved quality of life	Low-glycemic-index diet
Improved mood and self-esteem	High-protein diet

Source: https://www.ncbi.nlm.nih.gov/pubmed/23420000

From what I've seen at my nutrition practice, clients who limit their intake of simple sugars, refined carbohydrates, and saturated fats, and increased their slow digesting, complex carbohydrates, and low-glycemic-index foods (see page 118) were able to make this type of diet pattern more sustainable, all while managing their PCOS too. So, it doesn't matter necessarily how you lose the weight, just do what feels best, feels realistic and is the most sustainable for you!

DO I REALLY HAVE TO EXERCISE?

Exercising offers a host of benefits such as enhanced mood, improved stress management, decreased blood sugar, and increased insulin sensitivity. And who doesn't feel better after a great workout? Don't get stuck in the same spinning or weight-lifting routine, change it up! Combined exercise, such as switching between aerobic and resistance training, has shown greater benefits in PCOS management than just doing aerobic or resistance exercise alone.[103]

---

102   https://www.ncbi.nlm.nih.gov/pubmed?term=12574218
103   https://www.ncbi.nlm.nih.gov/pubmed/21431832

Total accumulated activity time has been shown to be even more beneficial to improving insulin sensitivity than the intensity of exercise alone. Therefore, no need to squeeze in a reckless 10-minute workout; moderate or even light activity for longer periods of time is good, nay, is great for your health! And, yes, even yoga counts. Women with excess body fat around the waist who went to three 1-hour yoga sessions weekly for a year showed decreased inflammation around the midsection–a common characteristic for women with PCOS. So, as you can see, there are many health perks to exercising lightly, moderately, or intensely–whatever works best for YOU!

Now that you know all the incredible benefits that exercising has to offer you in your PCOS management, the hardest part should be deciding what Rihanna smash hit you want to listen to while at the gym!

GOALS FOR EXERCISE:

1. Consider daily total movement and activity (walking, stairs) rather than intensity of exercise.

2. Only do exercise classes or programs that you enjoy.

3. Exercise between 45 to 60 minutes/day at least 4x week.

4. Switch up your exercise routines from aerobics to weight training to HIIT to yoga.

5. Remember, any exercise is better than no exercise! Work your way up from your baseline (yes, it's okay if your baseline is 0) in a slow, safe, and pragmatic fashion.

ADDED SUGAR + FIBER

Don't worry, you aren't crazy for craving carbs like ALL THE TIME when you have PCOS. In PCOS, strong cravings can be contributed to the spillover of the powerful hormone insulin, which is why you long for sweets and may have an appetite like The Hulk! Excess insulin is also why it's hard for women with PCOS to lose weight. Plus, high levels of androgens in PCOS have been associated with more carb cravings–this vicious cycle of craving carbs, eating carbs, crashing, then craving carbs again and again can be detrimental for blood sugar control as well as weight loss–gee thanks, insulin!

When it comes to PCOS management, choosing foods low in added sugars is important for both short-term and long-term health. The difference between added sugar and natural sugar is that added sugars are ADDED to foods while natural sugars are NATURALLY found in foods. Sorry to break it to you but added sugars in foods like candies, cookies, and sodas aren't found naturally. However, foods like fruits, vegetables, and milk naturally contain sugars. For instance, milk contains lactose, and fruit contains fructose and sucrose, all naturally occurring sugars. Added sugars, like white refined sugar or syrups, lack any real nutrients and can drastically contribute to weight gain and poor health outcomes.

No matter how you slice it, all added sugars are essentially equal from a nutritional perspective so portion control still matters. Therefore, you shouldn't squeeze the container of honey aimlessly on your oatmeal or dump all the brown sugar in your coffee in the world just because it's more natural.

The US Dietary Guidelines recommend our added sugar intake stay below 10% of calories, which is the equivalent of less than 50 grams, or 12.5 teaspoons, of added sugar per day if you eat a 2,000-calorie diet.[104] The American Heart Association recommends way less, aiming for 25 grams or 6 teaspoons (or 2 tablespoons) per day.

I'm definitely not saying to cut out carbohydrates completely, because that's not an effective or realistic long-term treatment for curbing cravings and managing PCOS. I'm saying let's find the best carbs to sprinkle your life with. And those are rich in a nondigestible form of carbohydrate known as fiber! Fiber does not spike your blood sugar and can even help to better regulate it. Fiber-rich foods also have a low GI. Foods with a low glycemic index tend to release glucose slowly into the blood, which is extremely beneficial to your health as well as blood sugar and insulin regulation.

Though numerous studies have shown the benefits of eating foods with a low GI to help improve insulin sensitivity in other chronic diseases (such as diabetes and heart disease), there isn't a general consensus at this time that a low GI diet will specifically treat PCOS. However, a low GI diet has been shown to have the following benefits on the symptoms associated with PCOS:

- Helpful in the management of PCOS by improving insulin sensitivity.

- May be useful for the lean PCOS population for whom weight loss is not needed but insulin needs to be better controlled, or in overweight patients for whom weight loss remains challenging

---

104 https://health.gov/dietaryguidelines/2015/resources/DGA_Cut-Down-On-Added-Sugars.pdf

- Can regulate menstruation. A systematic review showed that a low-glycemic-index weight-loss diet increased menstrual regularity for 95% of women compared to a standard weight-loss diet.[105]

- Can contribute to a greater improvement in emotions and quality of life compared to a healthy weight-loss diet.

The bottom line is that we know that whole grain, fiber-rich, low-sugar, and low-glycemic foods can reduce cravings and manage blood sugar. I believe the following strategies can boost your health, help you add more fiber, and improve your PCOS:

1. Add fruits, like blueberries, pears, and strawberries, and nuts and seeds into your morning Greek yogurt parfait.

2. Swap out mayo for avocado to get more belly-filling fiber.

3. Choose whole grain breads over wheat breads for additional fiber-rich benefits.

4. Use a variety of unique whole grains in your cooking, like farro, wheat berries, amaranth, sorghum, buckwheat, and quinoa.

5. Instead of refined white pasta, use whole grain or even bean-based pasta (such as Banza).

6. Swap out brown rice or white rice and use cauliflower or broccoli rice as your base.

7. In your morning smoothie, blend flaxseeds or oats for more fiber.

8. Sprinkle walnuts, hazelnuts, or chia seeds onto your salads instead of croutons.

---

105   https://www.ncbi.nlm.nih.gov/pubmed/23420000

9. Opt for lettuce or cabbage wraps instead of using buns at your next BBQ.

10. When baking, use whole wheat flour, oat flour, or almond flour instead of all-purpose white flour.

ADDED SUGARS	NATURAL SUGARS
Cookies	Fruits
Soda	Vegetables
Candy	Milk
Fruit juices	Dairy
Ketchup	
Flavored yogurt	
Pasta sauces	
Crackers	
Sweet drinks (flavored coffee, lemonade, sweetened tea, sports drinks)	

Sneaky Names of Added Sugar

- Brown sugar
- Coconut sugar
- Fructose
- Glucose
- Confectioners powdered sugar
- Sucrose
- Cane sugar
- Beet sugar
- High-fructose corn syrup
- Caramel
- Corn sweetener
- Honey
- Agave
- Invert sugar
- Molasses
- Any syrup (brown rice, malt, corn)

1. Become aware of sugar sources, sneaky names for sugar, and which products contain added sugars.

2. Track your food intake through an app such as MyFitnessPal or Fooducate to learn where those sneaky sources of added sugar are hanging out.

3. Be mindful of your treats. Choose desserts because they are special, not just because it's a basic Wednesday.

4. Keep fruits and vegetables readily accessible in your home so you aren't aimlessly munching on chips, cookies, or crackers that could have added sugar.

5. Before it's on the table, read the label. Because added sugar and natural sugars aren't separated on a food label yet (hopefully by 2020 though!), take a peek at the ingredient list.

6. Just because a product says "no added sugar" doesn't mean it's 100% pure. Food companies can add "fruit juice concentrate" or "fruit juice puree" and still label it "no added sugar." Also, if a recipe says "healthy" it still may have agave or honey in it, which is still considered added sugar.

7. Don't drink your sugar! Sugar sweetened beverages (SSB) like soda, juice, or energy drinks are the largest source of added sugars in the American diet. They make up almost half of the added sugars in our diet. SSB are linked to weight gain and adverse cardiometabolic health. Plus, studies have found that people who regularly consumed artificially sweetened beverages had a higher risk for health issues like weight gain, obesity, diabetes, and heart disease.[106] Therefore, the use of plain, unsweetened, carbonated water is strongly encouraged by the American Heart Association. Opt for unsweetened teas, seltzers, or infused water to help cut back on SSB.

8. Work with a health care professional to get the most individual type of education, care, and treatment.

OMEGA-3S

You better believe that because of their powerful health properties, omega-3s play a special role in managing PCOS. Omega-3s can help improve insulin sensitivity by breaking down that tough and strong insulin resistance. In 2018, a systematic review and meta-analysis showed that omega-3 fatty acids may be effective and safe for patients with PCOS with insulin resistance as well as high cholesterol, high LDL, and triglycerides. The long-term benefits of omega-3 supplementation is less certain but a short term (three-to six-month use) is recommended.

MAGNESIUM

Calling all dark chocolate lovers! You have officially been granted permission to eat that dark chocolate bar that's been calling your name for hours. Those with PCOS have been shown to have reduced levels of magnesium. In fact, being magnesium deficient puts you at 19 times higher risk of developing PCOS than those who have adequate magnesium.[107] Dark chocolate (aim for 85% cacao or higher) will help to restore your magnesium levels in no time.

---

106   http://www.cmaj.ca/content/189/28/E929
107   https://www.researchgate.net/publication/51241380_Serum_magnesium_concentrations_in_polycystic_ovary_syndrome_and_its_association_with_insulin_resistance

Additionally, magnesium has been shown to help regulate glucose and insulin. It's important to eat enough magnesium-rich foods because insulin resistance can negatively impact the absorption of magnesium, causing you to be even more prone to a deficiency. On the psychological front, anxiety is a very common symptom of PCOS. Menstrual problems, fertility issues, negative body image, and hirsutism are characteristics that can lead to anxiety in women with PCOS. Plus, anxiety and stress chip away at magnesium levels, leaving you further in the red. Fortunately, magnesium supplementation may help to combat feelings of anxiety and intense pressure. In addition, I urge you to talk openly in a clinical setting to a psychotherapist or mental health professional to learn how to keep your mind calm and cared for during this journey.

See Chapter 5, Premenstrual Disorders, for magnesium recommendations.

CALCIUM + VITAMIN D

Vitamin D and calcium play center stage in the role of PCOS management. Research shows a surprising 67% to 85% of women with PCOS are deficient in both vitamin D and calcium.[108] In fact, a deficiency in these two nutrients could even be a potent predictor of PCOS, *yikes!* Vitamin D is needed for proper calcium absorption, which underscores the importance of getting enough vitamin D in your diet.

Vitamin D and calcium may also help to keep inflammation at bay in PCOS patients. In a randomized, double-blind, placebo-controlled trial, vitamin D and calcium supplements helped reduce inflammation more than a placebo.[109] Taking vitamin D with calcium and metformin,

---

108   Ibid.
109   https://www.ncbi.nlm.nih.gov/pubmed/26119844

a common diabetes medication used in PCOS treatment, had more significant improvements for hirsutism, menstrual regularity, and ovulation, than metformin alone.[110] Plus, research has also linked vitamin D supplementation to reducing inflammation caused by insulin resistance.[111] So, make sure to get enough vitamin D and calcium to promote better PCOS management, stat!

DASH Diet

The Dietary Approach to Stop Hypertension (DASH) diet may be beneficial for PCOS patients. The DASH diet emphasizes foods that help to reduce high blood pressure, such as fruits, vegetables, low-fat dairy, fish, and whole grains. Overweight and obese subjects who followed the DASH diet for eight weeks showed beneficial effects on weight, BMI, triglycerides, LDL, and insulin compared to the control group. The array of antioxidants, magnesium, calcium, potassium, and dietary fiber coming from the DASH diet may be beneficial in those with PCOS to help control elevated levels of lipids and inflammation.

INOSITOL

Inositol, commonly known as myoinositol (MI) and d-chiro inositol (DI), is a B vitamin that supports cycle regularity, hormonal function, and balance. Inositol helps insulin become more sensitive and less "resistant." Just like you've talked to your partner about becoming

110   https://www.ncbi.nlm.nih.gov/pubmed/25535503
111   https://www.ncbi.nlm.nih.gov/pubmed/22780885

more sensitive with their emotions and less tough, inositol is trying to also trying to break down those walls with insulin.

As a supplement, MI may help to restore hormonal and reproductive balance, particularly in women with PCOS. Because it's generally safe and relatively inexpensive, it could be a good treatment in PCOS. A meta-analysis showed MI may help improve insulin regulation. In addition, SHBG (sex hormone binding globulin) is usually low in PCOS, and SHBG was restored back to normal after supplementation with MI for 24 weeks.[112]

In 2018, a meta-analysis concluded that inositol appears to regulate menstrual cycles, improve ovulation, and induce favorable metabolic changes in PCOS; however more evidence is needed for its impact on pregnancy and fertility.[113] Clearly, this is a buzzworthy topic so more conclusive research is likely going to escalate in the next few years. If this is something that interests you, keep an eye out on the research and as always, consult with your MD.

N-ACETYL CYSTEINE (NAC)

This may sound intimidating but N-acetyl cysteine is an antioxidant and amino acid worth talking about. NAC is the supplement form whereas cysteine is an amino acid form found in foods. NAC may have the ability to improve insulin in women with PCOS. NAC is craved by the body in order to produce and replenish an all-star antioxidant known as glutathione. Glutathione is the mecca of antioxidants and helps to reduce harmful oxidative stress, create a healthy immune system, and create a better reproductive environment. The more NAC you get, the more glutathione you have working its magic in your body. Seems like an easy win!

112   https://www.ncbi.nlm.nih.gov/pmc/articles/PMC5655679/#bib36
113   https://www.ncbi.nlm.nih.gov/pubmed/28544572

In a randomized clinical controlled trial, NAC supplementation was shown to have significant improvements in ovulation as well as pregnancy compared to a placebo.[114] Although research has only been conducted on NAC supplementation, it's recommended to eat a diet with a variety of cysteine-rich foods such as eggs, cod, chicken, sunflower seeds, cheese, lentils, salmon, and legumes. Recommended doses for NAC are between 1.3 to 6 grams per day.

TRACY'S TOP 10 TIPS FOR PCOS

1. Choose low-glycemic carbohydrates to decrease insulin production, such as sweet potato, brown rice, and quinoa.

2. Add proteins and fats to every meal to stay fuller longer and stop the rise in blood sugar levels, which results in less insulin stimulation.

3. Keep added sugars and refined carbohydrates to a minimum to dampen insulin spikes.

4. Go for fiber-rich foods to blunt blood sugar spikes and help to lower cholesterol.

5. Reduce saturated and trans fats to better manage PCOS, and opt for fatty acids and omega-3 unsaturated fats to help improve insulin resistance. Better yet, boost your omega-3s from food sources such as flaxseeds, avocados, salmon, or olive oil to get a bunch of inflammation-fighting compounds.

---

114   https://www.ncbi.nlm.nih.gov/pubmed/25653680

6. Add antioxidant-rich foods to reduce inflammation, like tomato, onions, butternut squash, and kale.

7. Eat calcium- and vitamin D-rich foods like yogurt, eggs, broccoli, and salmon.

8. Let magnesium be your friend. Add foods like dark chocolate, oysters, and beans into your life.

9. Don't be scared of carbohydrates. Simply add healthy fat and protein to minimize the potential blood sugar spike. For example, with a sweet potato, add a healthy fat like some olive oil and a protein like halibut so the sweet potato's ability to elevate blood sugar becomes greatly reduced. Try the sweet potato recipes on pages 199, 221, 230, 240, and 244.

10. Log the foods you eat on an app for one week to see exactly where your calories and added sugars are coming from, and scale back as needed to help with weight loss or blood sugar control. Work with a professional for support and guidance.

Five Foods for PCOS-Related Symptoms

These are my fave five foods to help manage PCOS-related symptoms, one bite at a time!

1. SWEET POTATOES: Don't restrict your carb intake entirely because it may cause bigger issues in your body when carbohydrates are eventually reintroduced (did someone say birthday cake?!)! Instead, choose the right type of carbohydrates for your body. The sweet potato is a great example of a complex, slow-releasing carbohydrate.

2. BEANS: Just like the sweet potato, beans are full of fiber, which means they are a slow-releasing carbohydrate that enable you to sustain longer periods of energy. Eating the right type of carbs, like beans, may even improve insulin sensitivity so remember to choose low-glycemic, complex carbohydrates throughout the day!

3. EGGS: Eggs are an essential and complete protein source because they contain all the amino acids your body can't produce on its own. Eggs have 0 grams of sugar and 0 carbohydrates so no need to worry about eggs sending glucose soaring. Plus, eggs may even have the ability to speed up metabolism. Choose organic eggs, or even omega-3-enriched eggs, when possible to prevent excess estrogen and antibiotics found in lots of conventionally raised animal products.

4. AVOCADOS: Healthy fats like avocados are vital in order to achieve optimal nutrient status and keep your blood sugar stable. Monounsaturated and polyunsaturated fats help process and digest vitamins, protect your organs, and even help regulate your body temperature. They contain antioxidant-rich vitamin A and E and may be able to help protect your eyes from harmful blue lights coming from your phone, tablet, and TV screen.

5. NUT BUTTERS: Nut butters (almond, peanut, cashew, hazelnut, etc.) or even seed butters (pumpkin, sunflower, sesame, etc.) are nutrient powerhouses. They are high in fiber, protein, magnesium, vitamin B, and immune-boosting vitamin E. You'll actually be full after eating this healthy fat and you will get a nice dose of satisfying protein too!

Glycemic Index Foods

The glycemic index (GI)[115, 116] is a value assigned to a food based on how fast or slow it can increase blood sugar. A food with a high GI raises blood sugar faster than a food with a lower GI. Aiming for low glycemic index foods are best to help manage blood sugar. These are the scores and categories:

- Low glycemic index = 0 to 55: Best to choose from this column
- Medium glycemic index = 56 to 70
- High glycemic index = 71 to 100

---

115   http://www.glycemicindex.com/foodSearch.php
116   https://www.nal.usda.gov/fnic/carbohydrates

FOOD	LOW GI 0 TO 55	MEDIUM GI 56 TO 70	HIGH GI 71 TO 100
Grains, breads, and cereals; nuts; legumes	Pumpernickel bread Grain bread 100% whole wheat bread Oatmeal (rolled or steel cut) Legumes Lentils Muesli Barley Whole grain spaghetti Chickpeas Black beans Cashews Hummus	Pita bread Quick oats Brown rice Couscous Corn tortilla Udon noodles	White bread Bagel Cornflakes Rice crackers Instant oatmeal Pretzels Rice cakes Rice milk Vanilla wafers
Fruit	Apples Oranges Banana Grapefruit Grapes Dried apricots Strawberries	Raisins Pineapple Cantaloupe Figs Dates	Watermelon Lychee
Vegetables	Carrots Sweet corn Sweet potato Parsnips Peas	Beets Russet potato (with skin)	Instant mashed potato
Other	Milk (full fat, soy, skim) Yogurt Chocolate	Honey Popcorn	Tofu-based frozen dessert

ENDOMETRIOSIS

Endometriosis is a chronic, inflammatory disease occurring when uterine lining cells and tissue that typically grows inside the uterus mistakenly grows outside of the uterus. This misplaced tissue can decide to grow anywhere in the pelvic cavity, such as in the fallopian tubes, bladder, ovaries, or even in the bowel. Just like the tissue normally regenerating in the uterus every month during a cycle, the misplaced tissue also responds to hormones and builds and sheds each month. However, the blood can't escape directly through the uterus and shed inside of the body, resulting in massive pain, inflammation, bowel issues, scar tissue, and even infertility.

HOW DO I KNOW
IF HAVE IT?

The exact cause of endometriosis remains unknown at this time. Hormonal, retrograde menstruation (or blood flowing back into the body instead of out of the body during a period), immune, inflammatory, anatomic, and genetic causes are partially to blame. If your mom or sister has endometriosis, you are more likely to have it. Another cause is high levels of prostaglandins, omega-6 fatty acid pro-inflammatory compounds, that can contribute to cramps and pain. Elevated levels of estrogen from chemicals such as polychlorinated biphenyls (PCBs) in the environment, endocrine disruptors such as parabens and phthalates, or through high consumption of meat, liver, and dairy are also risk factors.[117]

Endometriosis is an estrogen-dominant condition that occurs in 1 out of 10 women.[118]

A very common symptom of endometriosis is dysmenorrhea, pain associated with menstruation, as well as pain at other times throughout the month and during sex. Some may have debilitating pain and major discomfort, preventing them from engaging in typical day-to-day activities. On the other hand, some can go undiagnosed for most of their lives because they don't experience pain or any out-of-the-norm symptoms. Endometriosis is a leading cause of infertility and it's common for women to not know they have endometriosis until they have difficulty getting pregnant.

Talk to your doc! Explain the specifics and duration of your symptoms. If there aren't any glaring symptoms, bring up abnormal cycles or difficulties getting pregnant. The golden standard for confirming a diagnosis is through a laparoscopic procedure, a minimally invasive surgery used to examine the organs inside the abdomen.

WHAT DO I DO NOW?

Medication, surgery, and adjusting the diet are usually the winning combinations of treatment. As far as the diet, your nutrition goals

117   https://www.ncbi.nlm.nih.gov/pubmed/28326519
118   https://www.endofound.org/endometriosis-a-to-z

are to reduce already-elevated estrogen levels while sprinkling healthy antioxidants to combat inflammation. If you don't have endometriosis, you can still lower your risk by consuming a diet full of fruits and vegetables, dairy rich in calcium and vitamin D, fish oils, and omega-3 fatty acids.

WHAT ELSE DOES THE SCIENCE SAY?

One study showed that women who ate foods high in fat (particularly trans fats, mea, and dairy) as well as red beef (such as pork and ham), and who drank alcohol were all at higher risk for getting endometriosis.[119]

- Cut out trans fats and focus more on moderate to low intakes of plant-based healthy fats such as nuts, seeds, olive oil, walnut oil, or avocado oil.

- Swap your red beef for heart-healthy fish or plant-based proteins, and try to eat grass-fed and certified organic meats when possible, no more than two servings per week.

- Aim for moderate to low alcohol intake per week (one to two servings per week).

Saturated fat has been shown to increase estrogen in premenopausal women.[120]

- Keep saturated fat intake moderate to low to control excess estrogen levels. Be mindful of saturated fat coming from butter, oils, cheese, milk, red meat, and coconut-based products.

---

119   https://www.ncbi.nlm.nih.gov/pubmed/28326519
120   https://www.ncbi.nlm.nih.gov/pubmed/22399233

- Aim for lean proteins with minimal to no saturated fat such as high-quality, skinless poultry, turkey, or omega-3-enriched eggs no more than five times per week.

- Opt for more plant-based proteins like beans, quinoa, lentils, and chickpea pasta four to five times per week for a dose of calcium, potassium, and magnesium, all which can help with painful cramps.

Vitamin B6 is extremely useful; it can help excess estrogen become inactive and creates more anti-inflammatory compounds, known as gamma linolenic acid (GLA), which can help inhibit the growth of endometrial tissue.

- Eat more vitamin B6 to create more anti-inflammatory GLA such as eggs, oatmeal, and wheat germ, and eat more GLA-rich foods like hemp seeds, oats, spirulina, and barley.

Thiamine (vitamin B1), folate, vitamin C, and vitamin E solely from food sources (not from supplements) were shown to reduce endometriosis risk. Women with the most intakes of each of those nutrients lowered the chances of endometriosis diagnosis.[121]

- Eat foods with folate, such as fortified cereals, adzuki beans, mung beans, and chickpeas and thiamine-rich foods, such as oranges, oats, and sunflower seeds. Don't forget to add broccoli, nut butters, and strawberries to your diet for a boost of vitamin C.

Women who had surgery for endometriosis received vitamins A, C, E, and B6, and the minerals calcium, magnesium, selenium, zinc, and iron, as well as omega-3s and omega-6s for six months post op. They found significant improvements in overall health and quality of life after taking vitamins vs. placebo.[122]

121   https://www.ncbi.nlm.nih.gov/pmc/articles/PMC3916184
122   https://www.ncbi.nlm.nih.gov/pubmed/17434511

- Consider a multivitamin with vitamins A, C, E, and B6, calcium, magnesium, selenium, zinc, and iron, and high-quality fish oil (omega-3 and omega-6) supplements.

There is no definitive connection between the occurrence of endometriosis and caffeine.

- Consume coffee in moderation and modify accordingly.

In 2018, a large meta-analysis and systematic review found dietary isoflavones were linked to a reduction in endometrial cancer risk in both Asian and non-Asian countries. In fact, isoflavone intake from soy products and legumes lowered the risk of endometrial cancer by 19%.[123] Another meta-analysis found that soy isoflavone intakes were unrelated to estrogen levels in premenopausal women.[124]

- No need to stay clear from isoflavones (like edamame, tofu, or soy milk) or soy products. Just eat organic and in moderation!
- Rewire eating habits if you have endometriosis to have more veggies, more omega-3, less caffeine, less red meat, less alcohol, and less trans fat.

REDUCE GLUTEN—ONLY IF YOU HAVE SYMPTOMS

In the world of nutrition, gluten's relation to the prevention and management of endometriosis is debatable. For some, gluten, a protein found in wheat, may not bother their pelvic symptoms. For others, gluten may make them feel pretty awful. Although not widely researched, a small study consisting of 207 women with

123   https://www.ncbi.nlm.nih.gov/pubmed/27914914
124   https://www.ncbi.nlm.nih.gov/pubmed/19299447

endometriosis found that 75% of women reported statistically significant improvements in painful symptoms after going gluten-free for 12 months. Improvements were seen in general health, social functioning, and mental health. In fact, no patients reported worsening of pain by going gluten-free. Therefore, it could be recommended for some to go gluten-free to lessen symptoms of endometriosis.[125]

If gluten seems to be upsetting digestion, increasing pelvic pain, and triggering an uncomfortable autoimmune response, avoid gluten for a few weeks to months and then reassess your symptoms. What do you have to lose?

CUT BACK ON RED MEAT

Studies have shown that limiting red meat consumption may be advisable for women with endometriosis, *particularly those who experience painful endometriosis-related symptoms.*[126] Eating red meat, particularly those with added hormones, has been linked to elevated estrogen, which doesn't favor a calm, cool environment in the body.

As women increased their red meat intake (both processed and unprocessed), so did their risk for developing endometriosis. Those who ate more than two servings of red meat per day had a 56% higher risk of endometriosis when compared to those who had one or less servings of red meat per week. Eating ham, beef, pork, and other kinds of meat was connected with higher endometriosis risk,

---

125   https://www.ncbi.nlm.nih.gov/pubmed/23334113
126   https://www.ncbi.nlm.nih.gov/pubmed/29870739

whereas eggs, poultry, fish, shellfish, and even butter (surprisingly!) were not related to endometriosis risk.[127, 128]

Beyond endometriosis, the consumption of red meat has been linked to the development of devastating diseases such as diabetes, cardiovascular disease, and cancer. Red meat may increase estrogen levels as a result of eating hormone-treated animals. Added hormones in the diet from animal products like red meat may foster the development of pro-inflammatory cytokines, which possibly enhances inflammation associated with endometriosis. By decreasing estrogen and inflammatory prostaglandins levels through informed food choices, you may help to shrink the inflammatory nature of endometriosis. In fact, women with dysmenorrhea reported less pain by eating a low-fat vegetarian diet. So, swapping out high-fat meat for low-fat veggies could be the ultimate recipe for those with pain.[129]

INCREASE OMEGA-3s

Painful periods and generalized pelvic pain are common symptoms in endometriosis. It's like lighting a candle from both ends when you combine the inflammatory nature of endometriosis with the inflammatory prostaglandins (aka fat cells) released from the uterus during a period. Keep the pain to a minimum by eating vibrant fruits and vegetables and anti-inflammatory omega-3s to help uncomfortable spasms and cramps.

Taking omega-3 fish oil (known as EPA + DHA) and eating omega-3-rich food and more anti-inflammatory foods has been

127   https://www.ncbi.nlm.nih.gov/pubmed/15254009
128   https://www.ncbi.nlm.nih.gov/pubmed/29870739
129   https://www.ncbi.nlm.nih.gov/pubmed/10674588

associated with reduced inflammation, painful periods, and dysmenorrhea.[130, 131] In fact, eating more omega-3 fatty acids was linked to a 22% decrease in the rate of endometriosis diagnosis.[132] Even more reason to start swapping your beef entree for omega-3-rich salmon, mackerel, or oysters! Aim to have three to five servings of fish per week.

Eat a ratio of 3:1 omega-3s to omega-6s. That means there should be more omega-3s in your diet such as salmon, walnuts, spinach, and chia seeds than omega-6s such as pistachios and pine nuts.

INCREASE ANTIOXIDANTS

When assessing the best diet to help manage endometriosis, a comprehensive study showed that women with endometriosis boosted their health by eating a diet rich in antioxidants, mainly fueled by plants. Eating more plant foods rich in vitamin C and especially vitamin E may be helpful in reducing the growth of injured and inflamed endometrial tissue and cells, which may help ease the pain associated with endometriosis.[133, 134]

Plus, magnesium-rich foods like almonds, bananas, and Swiss chard can help to relax smooth muscle contraction from the uterus to help relieve pelvic pain.

PSA: It goes without saying that smokers are more susceptible to worsening inflammation, cellular damage, and oxidative stress, all of which don't prioritize healing and reparation in the body.

130 https://www.ncbi.nlm.nih.gov/pubmed/29870739
131 https://www.ncbi.nlm.nih.gov/pubmed/23642910
132 https://www.ncbi.nlm.nih.gov/pmc/articles/PMC3916184/#R8
133 https://www.ncbi.nlm.nih.gov/pmc/articles/PMC3916184
134 https://doi.org/10.1186/1477-7827-7-54

There is a strong link between oxidative stress, in the form of cellular or tissue damage, and in the development of endometriosis.[135] In fact, low zinc has been associated with increased inflammation in women with endometriosis.

- A diet bountiful with antioxidants helps to repair damaged cells and keep inflammation under control. Eat at least four servings of vegetables and one serving of fruit per day.
- Aim for at least three colors per meal.
- Vitamin E from food sources was associated with the largest reduction of endometriosis risk in research. The two richest sources in the study were peanut butter and vegetable oils (sunflower, corn oil, soybean).[136, 137] Other vitamin E-rich foods are sunflower seeds, hazelnuts, and almonds.
- Eat vitamin A-rich foods such as squash, sweet potato, carrots, spinach, and dandelion greens.
- Eat vitamin C-rich food such as citrus, broccoli, kale, and strawberries.
- Eat iron-rich fruits and vegetables to replenish the high amount of blood loss during a period and to combat tiredness. Iron-rich fruits are apricots, goji berries, and raisins. Spirulina, seaweed, mushrooms, and potatoes are also sources of iron-rich veggies.
- To achieve hormonal balance, minimize pesticide and hormone disruptors by purchasing organically grown produce when possible. Pesticides can reduce the antioxidants in produce so follow the Environmental Working Group List for which produce you should buy organic vs. conventional. Additionally, opt for organic (dairy, eggs, poultry, fish, butter, etc.) when possible.

---

135   https://www.hindawi.com/journals/omcl/2017/7265238/
136   https://www.ncbi.nlm.nih.gov/pubmed/2520267
137   https://www.ncbi.nlm.nih.gov/pubmed/28326519

2019 Environmental Working Group List
(USDA, www.ewg.org)

DIRTY DOZEN	CLEAN FIFTEEN
Strawberries	Avocado
Spinach	Sweet corn
Kale	Pineapple
Nectarines	Frozen sweet peas
Apples	Onions
Grapes	Papaya
Peaches	Eggplant
Cherries	Asparagus
Pears	Kiwi
Tomatoes	Cabbage
Celery	Cauliflower
Potatoes	Cantaloupe
	Broccoli
	Mushrooms
	Honeydew

UP THE VITAMIN D AND CALCIUM

This nutritional dynamic duo is back at it, now showcasing their strengths by helping to reduce endometriosis risk and helping to manage and heal symptoms. In a study of 700,000 women, intakes of milk and other low-fat dairy foods were associated with a lower risk of endometriosis. Women eating more than three servings of dairy per day were 18% less likely to be diagnosed with endometriosis than those who had two servings per day. Plus, women with high levels of vitamin D were associated with a 24% lower risk of endometriosis than women with the lowest concentration of vitamin D.[138]

That being said, there is no reason to eliminate dairy from your diet if you have endometriosis. For those who want to keep their risk of endometriosis as low as possible, sprinkle in more vitamin D and calcium throughout the day. Switch to organic, low-fat dairy products to limit your exposure to hormones added to food, aiming for at least three servings per day. Start your day with Greek yogurt and almonds with berries, have a vegetable egg frittata made with a splash of milk with Parmesan, kale, mushrooms, and broccoli for lunch, and end your day with salmon, sweet potato, and asparagus for a day loaded to the brim with vitamin D and calcium.

ESTROGEN SQUASHERS

To ensure estrogen levels are A-OK in the body and not surging like that pricey Uber ride on New Year's Eve, here are some tips to keep it balanced.

- Indole-3-carbinol is a compound found in cruciferous vegetables that enhances the metabolism and breakdown of estrogen. Eat at least 1 cup a day of these crunchy and helpful veggies such as Brussels sprouts, broccoli, kale, radishes, cabbage, and cauliflower.

- Folate, vitamin B6, and vitamin B12 are all involved in estrogen metabolism and more importantly, excess estrogen detoxification and removal. Therefore, it's essential to eat enough of these vitamins to minimize your risk of increased estrogen lurking in the bod.

138   https://www.ncbi.nlm.nih.gov/pubmed/23380045

- Those who ate a diet rich in fat and low in fiber had too much of a harmful gut bacteria enzyme hanging out, known as beta-glucuronidase. In order to sweep this enzyme from the gut and clear the intestinal pathway for the removal of excess estrogen and other toxins, eat veggies like collard greens, kale, eggplant, asparagus, and potato. In general, plants and pre/probiotic-rich foods will keep your gut as clean as a whistle!

- Research suggests that phytoestrogens may help conditions associated with estrogen imbalances, such as PMS, endometriosis, and even menopausal symptoms.[139] Phytoestrogen-rich foods can mimic estrogen in the bod. Why is this important? Well, these foods produce "weak" estrogens when compared to the "strong" estrogens the body makes (coming from the ovaries, adrenal glands, and fat tissues). Weak estrogens from food may block "stronger" estrogen production, which in turn can help the body strike a better hormonal balance. Lignans found in fiber-rich foods, like flaxseeds, pumpkin seeds, berries, soy, legumes, and vegetables can help to reduce estrogen in the blood and keep estrogen balanced. In fact, researchers found that flaxseed bread may help to minimize breast tenderness associated with excess estrogen.

See Chapter 5, Premenstrual Disorders, for treatment ideas because most women with endometriosis tend to have PMS/PMDD.

139   https://www.ncbi.nlm.nih.gov/pubmed/9751507

THYROID DYSFUNCTION

The thyroid is a pretty powerful gland. Like a joystick, it controls our metabolism, body temperature, reproductive system, fertility, and even cycle regularity. The thyroid produces hormones, known as T3 and T4, that virtually affect every organ of the body. Your brain (specifically the hypothalamus-pituitary-thyroid axis) regularly surveys the body to see if it needs to make more or less hormones. It's like a great SoulCycle instructor that can always read the vibes in the room and decide whether to tell the class to add or remove resistance on the bike. They know what's best!

A bit more about the thyroid hormones, T3 and T4. T3 is the more powerful one, but 90% of the thyroid hormones floating around are actually T4. Because your body naturally has more T4, it is constantly converting T4 into T3 to balance things out. This conversion relies on a boatload of nutrients from your diet, such as zinc, iodine, and vitamin B12. So, if you have nutritional gaps in your diet, it's possible your thyroid hormones could be out of whack.

HYPOTHYROIDISM

An underactive, or sluggish, thyroid is one of the most common conditions I see at my nutrition practice. The majority of hypothyroidism cases are caused by Hashimoto's thyroiditis, or Hashimoto's disease, an autoimmune condition when your thyroid hormones accidentally attack your healthy thyroid gland.

In Hashimoto's disease, the thyroid gland is basically striking out, unable to produce enough thyroid hormones. Its peppy teammate, thyroid stimulating hormone (TSH), tries to rally the thyroid gland but ultimately fails. As a result, the thyroid becomes sluggish, you may feel off-kilter and have symptoms such as hair loss, weight gain, fatigue, or even infertility. You may also experience major PMS, low sex drive, or painful and heavy periods. Hashimoto's disease contributes to all of these not-so-great symptoms.

Imagine accidentally washing a red sock with your white clothes. Your white clothes will inadvertently turn pink as a repercussion, which is annoying, but there are solutions. The same goes for Hashimoto's disease—it doesn't mean to attack your thyroid and make you feel badly as an unfortunate side effect. Thankfully, there are some food fixes to remedy the situation.

HYPERTHYROIDISM

An overproduction of thyroid hormones is known as hyperthyroidism. Graves' disease is an autoimmune disorder that causes an overactive thyroid. Symptoms of hyperthyroidism include weight loss, hair loss, extreme hunger, frequent bowel movements, anxiety, and irritability.

HOW DID I GET IT?

Unfortunately, there isn't a clear reason for getting hyper- or hypothyroidism. Factors run the gamut and include genetics (70% to 80%), hormonal imbalances, existing autoimmune disorders, diabetes, environmental conditions, toxins, and iodine or other nutrient deficiencies.[140] Progesterone and estrogen have a tight-knit relationship with the thyroid gland. If either hormone becomes off-balance, so does the thyroid. Womp womp.

PROGESTERONE: Low progesterone can contribute to estrogen dominance and interfere with thyroid hormone balance. A deficiency in thyroid hormones has been related to a decrease in progesterone.

ESTROGEN: High estrogen and stress (aka cortisol) can block thyroid hormone production. Metabolism can slow down if thyroid hormones are blocked, which may cause fat storage and estrogen buildup.

> Chronic stress has the power to directly interfere with thyroid hormones that influence and control the menstrual cycle. So it bears repeating that it's essential to relax once in a while!

HOW DO I KNOW IF I HAVE THYROID ISSUES?

If you have out-of-the-norm symptoms or period woes, get thyroid labs (such T3, T4, TSH, TPO, thyroglobulin, or thyroid antibodies) tested by your doctor. Low thyroid hormones can negatively

140   https://www.ncbi.nlm.nih.gov/pubmed/16381988

impact sex hormones that affect your cycle and fertility. Menstrual problems (such as heavy or absent periods) are more common in those with hypothyroidism than in hyperthyroidism so it's important to find and treat the underlying cause of your cycle issues.

WHAT DO I EAT NOW?

The goal is to correct the autoimmune condition that lies underneath through the power of food. Nutrients can naturally support thyroid function, boost your immune system, and fix menstrual irregularities. Your diet should be full of whole foods like veggies, fruits, beans, lentils, healthy fats, omega-3s, legumes, and lean proteins. Reach for foods rich in vitamins A, C, B12, E, zinc, and selenium to support your thyroid and reproductive health. The less soda, processed foods, sugars, added fats, and meats, the better. Don't write off any food groups entirely from your diet before learning more about them, you could be nutritionally missing out!

IODINE

Iodine is like your thryoid's phone charger, you rely heavily on it. In the typical Western diet, we get plenty of iodine through food, which is fundamental because the body doesn't produce iodine. However, if you do not eat enough iodine-rich sources, just like your phone, your thyroid hormones too could be running out of battery.

Without thyroid hormones, you stand the chance of developing hypothyroidism, a sluggish metabolism, or a goiter (enlarged thyroid). Adding iodized salt to the diet may help improve cycle irregularity in women who were using little or no iodized salt.[141] If salt

---

141   https://www.ncbi.nlm.nih.gov/pubmed/8051643

isn't an appealing add-on, you can get iodine through food sources such as seaweed, shrimp, cheese, and tuna. Be sure to ask your doctor for a blood test to make sure your iodine levels are balanced.

CRUCIFEROUS VEGETABLES

Cruciferous vegetables (like kale, broccoli, or Brussels sprouts) naturally release goitrogens, a pesky compound that can block the thyroid from using iodine to produce hormones needed to regulate the menstrual cycle. If you have sufficient iodine and adequate thyroid hormones (either naturally or due to medication), you shouldn't have a problem. Plus, cooking cruciferous vegetables (instead of eating them raw) can diminish goitrogen effects.[142]

For someone with low thyroid hormones with hypothyroidism (and whose thyroid hormones are not medically managed), eating raw, cruciferous vegetables can send thyroid hormones further into a slump. That's why it's recommended to eat less than ½ cup of cooked cruciferous vegetables per day. If your treatment (such as medication) for hypothyroidism is working and your thyroid hormones are balanced, you can definitely eat as much cooked and raw veggies as you like.

> Eating raw, cruciferous vegetables doesn't directly cause thyroid issues so don't avoid these healthy, nutritional gems to keep your thyroid health intact. If you are worried, ask your doc to test your iodine, but otherwise, you have the green (and crunchy) light to eat all the veggies!

142   https://www.ncbi.nlm.nih.gov/pubmed/17343774

SOY

A hot topic, yes. Soy may have goitrogen effects (similar to those of cruciferous vegetables), which can lower thyroid hormone production. However, a review of 14 research studies found that soy protein and soy isoflavones, such as edamame, tofu, miso, and soy milk, had little to no effect on thyroid function in healthy people with adequate iodine levels.[143] Plus, researchers believe that soy intake doesn't cause hypothyroidism in people with adequate iodine.[144] So, there's no scientific validity to completely avoid soy foods if you have hypothyroidism, you are trying to reduce your risk of hypothyroidism, or you are on thyroid medication. Soy is absolutely fine to eat if you have a thyroid issue, especially if your iodine intake is adequate and your iodine levels are sufficient. Choose high-quality and organic soy products that have been minimally processed, and simply eat in moderation.

CALCIUM + VITAMIN D

Calcium is a very high-maintenance mineral. Striking the perfect calcium balance is more than just for good bone health; it's essential for reducing PMS, cycle regularity, and ensuring that our reproductive cells and hormones are communicating on the same Wi-Fi network. So many players are needed at bat to keep calcium levels balanced. Let's meet your hormonal lineup.

- Parathyroid hormone (PTH), a thyroid hormone that works closely with the bones to ensure calcium levels are sufficient.

143   https://www.uptodate.com/contents/thyroid-hormone-action/abstract/34
144   https://www.ncbi.nlm.nih.gov/pubmed/16571087

- Calcitonin, a hormone that regulates calcium blood levels.
- Vitamin D, a vitamin and an under-the-radar hormone, that maintains the concentration of calcium in the blood.

All of these hormones play a role in achieving the perfect calcium balance by acting on the bones, kidneys, and intestines. If low calcium is detected in the blood, an alarm goes off in the body and a cascade of events occur to take corrective measures. PTH takes charge and forages to find calcium through bone and kidney reabsorption, and increases the absorption of calcium in your intestines. After taking these steps to ensure calcium balance, the alarm stops ringing and calcium is no longer in the red, *phew*!

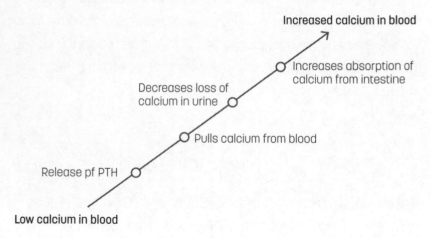

As far as vitamin D, did you know that it is responsible for activating and balancing thyroid hormones? Without enough vitamin D, our thyroids can't rise to the occasion. Those with hypothyroidism are often low in vitamin D and hyperthyroidism is associated with bone loss so we have to pick up the vitamin D slack in both thyroid conditions!

Calcium and vitamin D supplementation may be a helpful tool in reducing PMS-related symptoms such as irritability and depression in those with abnormal PTH levels.[145, 146] It may take a solid team (as you've learned from above) but maintaining good calcium and vitamin D balance in the body–either through foods or supplements–is essential to keeping our reproductive and thyroid health in check.

GLUTATHIONE + SELENIUM

This pair of aces are back at it again, protecting our reproductive and thyroid health with the attention it deserves. By eating the mineral selenium, our bodies get access to an exuberant and vibrant antioxidant, glutathione. Glutathione fights inflammation and has your health's best interest at heart. But how?

Well, both glutathione and selenium shield the thyroid from inflammation, which is especially helpful in those with Hashimoto's disease when the thyroid becomes inflamed. The benefits don't stop there. Selenium is also necessary for thyroid health because it aids in the conversion of thyroid hormones T4 to T3. This process re-energizes sluggish thyroid hormones, and can even improve the moods in those with Hashimoto's disease.[147] On top of that, research has shown that in Graves' disease, selenium supplementation improved thyroid functioning just after six months.[148]

In addition to the thyroid benefits, selenium promotes the development of mature follicles, nurturing them for a strong, healthy ovulation. So, keep this mineral in mind if babies are on the brain. Selenium is typically found in the soil but due to overuse of

---

145   https://www.ncbi.nlm.nih.gov/pubmed/17366354
146   https://www.ncbi.nlm.nih.gov/pubmed/9731851
147   https://www.ncbi.nlm.nih.gov/pubmed/20883174
148   https://www.ncbi.nlm.nih.gov/pubmed/30356415

farming and diminishing amounts in the ground, more people are susceptible to selenium deficiency. So, put this mineral at the top of your to-do list and aim to eat more selenium through Brazil nuts, eggs, sunflower seeds, legumes, chicken, and pork, or consider taking a supplement. Either way, your body will thank you.

ZINC

Spoiler alert: Zinc is basically the Wizard behind the curtain. Zinc operates a ton of controllers that impact our reproductive and thyroid health. As discussed in other chapters, we've learned that zinc can improve period pain, reduce inflammation, and even regulate our mentrual cycle. And when it comes to the thyroid, a zinc deficiency may result in low thyroid hormones, leading to diminished reproductive health and poor egg development. No thanks!

Just like iodine and selenium, zinc is able to power on thyroid hormones, which is essential in conditions like Hashimoto's disease that desperately need assistance with this process. In fact, zinc supplementation was able to increase thyroid hormone, T3, and successfully converted T4 to T3.[149] *Bonus:* the absorption of zinc in food becomes enhanced when thyroid hormones are balanced in the body.[150] Therefore, the thyroid and zinc relationship is a two-way street

Take this romance to the next level (go ahead, make it Instagram official) and eat plenty of zinc-rich foods such as pumpkin seeds, oysters, red meat, eggs, whole grains, asparagus, broccoli, shellfish

---

149   https://www.ncbi.nlm.nih.gov/pubmed/8157857
150   https://www.ncbi.nlm.nih.gov/pubmed/20688624

such as lobster or shrimp, and chicken. If you don't think you eat enough zinc, it may be time to add a regular supplement to your diet.

ALCOHOL

You may not realize that breaking down those spicy margaritas and bottles of vino in the body takes a lot of work. However, alcohol metabolism may actually prevent autoimmune disorders like Hashimoto's disease. A large study in Denmark found that the consumption of up to 10 glasses of wine per week had protective effects against the development of Hashimoto's disease.[151] Regardless if your thyroid is medically managed, please note that excessive alcohol intake may reduce the absorption of helpful vitamins and minerals, so enjoy a glass every now and then.

IRON

Iron is a must! It helps to create thyroid hormones and keeps them standing strong. Folks with Hashimoto's disease commonly experience fatigue and may also have stomach issues that decrease iron absorption. This double whammy coupled with expected blood loss during a period can further dip iron, which may subsequently send thyroid hormones crashing to the ground. A word to the wise would be not to neglect this powerful mineral!

Eating and rebuilding iron through animal- and plant-based sources can help you create an iron-proof vest, protecting you from any

---

151   https://www.ncbi.nlm.nih.gov/pubmed/22802427

roadblocks or deficiencies along the way. And remember, iron delivers energy-boosting oxygen to every single cell in the body, so you'll turn into the Energizer Bunny, stat! If you think your iron intake isn't up to par, get blood panels drawn (such as iron, ferritin, hemoglobin, hematocrit, transferrin, and total iron-binding capacity [TIBC]) to check for a possible imbalance.

Iron + Nonheme Iron

Vitamin C and iron (especially coming from plants) are like Tina Fey + Amy Poehler, total besties that make magic when working together. There are two forms of iron, heme and nonheme. Heme iron is more easily absorbed and mostly found in animal sources like red meat, oysters, chicken, and pork. Nonheme iron sources (such as tofu, pumpkin seeds, beans, lentils, and quinoa) is more stubborn and not as easily absorbed. Vitamin C enhances the absorption of nonheme food sources so the body can use it more easily, *no ifs, ands, or buts about it*. Next meal, pair vitamin C (tomato, lemon, peppers, kale, broccoli) with nonheme foods, deal?

GLUTEN UPDATE

Both Hashimoto's disease and Graves' disease are known as autoimmune diseases, conditions where your body attacks healthy cells by mistake. Do you know what also is an autoimmune disease? Celiac disease. In these folks, a protein found in wheat, known as gluten, sets off a chain of inflammatory reactions in the body, leading to gastrointestinal pain. To manage their condition, folks are advised to remove gluten from their diets and eat gluten-free.

Besides painful belly symptoms, people with celiac disease may not be able to absorb key nutrients like iron, zinc, or vitamin D, all of which are needed to facilitate a healthy menstrual cycle. These autoimmune conditions can cause major period woes like cramps and intense pain and negatively impact the cycle by messing with sex hormones, like progesterone, testosterone, and estrogen. In fact, those with Hashimoto's disease have a higher chance of menstrual disturbances (such as irregular, heavy, missing, or short periods), which can lead to fertility issues down the road.

Oddly enough, researchers have been intrigued by patients with both Hashimoto's disease and celiac disease. Studies have found that a gluten-free diet may bring clinical benefits to women (such as thyroid hormone regulation and improved vitamin D levels) with autoimmune thyroid diseases.[152] In simple terms, Hashimoto's disease patients may feel better after going gluten-free.

If you have Hashimoto's disease (regardless if you are being medically managed), you might want to try a gluten-free diet. Just make sure you aren't leaving any major nutritional holes in your diet, like a gap in B vitamins, iron, zinc, or magnesium. Work with a professional before going gluten-free to learn how to adjust your diet accordingly. After a few months, assess how you feel. As they say, the proof is in the (gluten-free) pudding.

---

152   https://www.ncbi.nlm.nih.gov/pubmed/30060266

9

AMENORRHEA

Amenorrhea is the absence of monthly periods; it's either on pause or permanently out of the office. Due to the stigma surrounding menstrual health, women are ashamed and aren't encouraged to openly talk about period woes, and this clinical problem can often go undiagnosed and untreated.

HOW DO I GET IT?

A wide range of factors and underlying health issues can impact a female's ability to maintain or even have a menstrual cycle. This very complex condition may be surprising to those who look like the ideal picture of health on the outside but whose reproductive health may be in need of serious attention. Numerous changes can occur in the hormones, glands, or organs involved in the menstrual cycle. Below are possible causes of amenorrhea:

- Chronic undernourishment
- Nutrient deficiencies
- Excessive exercise
- Extreme stress and anxiety
- Birth control, IUD, or post birth control syndrome
- Rapid weight loss

- Self-inflicted starvation
- Eating disorders such as anorexia nervosa, orthorexia, and drunkorexia
- Environmental stress or trauma
- Genetic abnormalities
- Issues with the pituitary gland and/or hypothalamus
- Excess prolactin and other hormonal imbalances
- Ovarian dysfunction or failure
- Delayed puberty
- Hypo- or hyperthyroidism
- Polycystic ovarian syndrome
- Breast feeding
- Pregnancy

Eating Disorders Old and New

Orthorexia is a newly coined eating pattern in which the obsession with health ultimately becomes unhealthy. It is defined as a fixation on only eating foods that are considered to be healthy, clean, and pure and often is coupled with avoidance of certain food groups as they are perceived by that person to be dangerous and bad. This is extremely common in hypothalamic amenorrhea (see page 147). Drunkorexia is another newly coined term for those women typically on college campuses, who save all calories for just alcohol in an effort to restrict calories/lose weight and have enhanced reaction to alcohol. Both eating patterns can compromise reproductive and menstrual cycle health.

WHAT WENT WRONG?

Everyone's brains are wired differently. You know your coworker who is always so cool, calm, and collected before a big presentation while you've sweat through your T-shirt and your deodorant just can't save you? Well, this is an example of how the brain and the nervous system causes individuals to react differently in the same environmental situation.

There should be a harmonious dance between the two nervous systems, known as the sympathetic (fight-or-flight hormones) and parasympathetic systems (rest-and-digest hormones). If they are represented equally in the brain, the menstrual cycle mostly remains unscathed from stress, exercise, weight loss, and so on. But that isn't the case for many of us. A ton of factors send the sympathetic nervous system into overdrive from intense working environments, vigorous exercise regimens, weight loss, and even bouts of mental and emotional stress. Although these circumstances are common in this day and age when our diet-obsessed, fast-paced culture is constantly preying upon us, they still have enough power to negatively influence our reproductive health.

LET'S BREAK IT DOWN

Amenorrhea can be broken down into two subcategories.

1. Primary amenorrhea, when a woman doesn't get her first period by the age of 16. Causes are sometimes unknown and can be difficult to treat.

2. Secondary amenorrhea, when a woman who once had regular cycles misses her period for three cycles in a row OR when a woman who had irregular cycles misses her period for more than six months. Causes are typically known and can be treated.

Hypothalamic amenorrhea (HA) is a form of secondary amenorrhea classified as stress-, weight-loss, or exercise-related amenorrhea.

MORE ABOUT HYPOTHALAMIC AMENORRHEA

At my nutrition practice, I've seen clients most commonly lose their periods because of HA, which accounts for more than 30% of amenorrhea cases in women of reproductive age.[153] Patients often have high stress, low estrogen, low insulin, low calorie intake, intense exercise patterns, thyroid dysfunction, or bone loss. These factors can wreak hormonal havoc, leading to imbalances in the backbones needed to support the menstrual cycle, like FSH, LH, and estrogen. HA can also significantly contribute to osteoporosis, ovary dysfunction, and difficulties getting pregnant down the road.

There is a lack of communication between the brain and the ovaries in HA. The part of your brain that controls reproduction and the menstrual cycle (known as the hypothalamic-pituitary-adrenal axis) can become suppressed in HA and stop firing a necessary hormone needed to menstruate (GnRH) if we eat too little, are too stressed or go to the gym too often. The body needs enough energy to produce a menstrual cycle so if the body becomes energy deficient (stemming from reduced food intake or strenuous exercise), it no longer has the stamina or fuel to menstruate.

153   https://www.ncbi.nlm.nih.gov/pubmed/4469672

Nutritional deficiencies can also cause HA. It's like your cell phone battery—it won't last the entire day when the battery percentage starts off at less than 5%. You have to charge your body with food the same way you have to charge your phone with a plug.

I had the privilege of listening to Dr. Jaime Knopman, a prestigious, New York City-based reproductive endocrinologist and fertility specialist at Colorado Center for Reproductive Medicine talk about menstrual and hormonal balance during a panel discussion in which she described hypothalamic amenorrhea from a musical perspective. She explained that the reproductive system works like an orchestra. The brain acts as the conductor and orders the instruments (organs like the thyroid and ovaries) on exactly what to do. In hypothalamic amenorrhea, the brain powers off so the instruments no longer have any direction, and the whole philharmonic subsequently shuts down.

Fortunately, you can take definitive actions and modify risk factors to reverse and prevent both hypothalamic amenorrhea (HA) and the female athlete triad.

FEMALE ATHLETE TRIAD

Female athlete triad is a syndrome describing the coexistence of three distinct medical conditions in athletic girls and women.

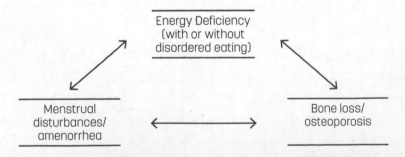

The female athlete triad is defined as energy deficiency, the loss or irregularity of a period, and low bone density or osteoporosis.

These three risk factors are especially crosslinked in female athletes and in non-athletic recreational exercisers, which is why it makes up a triangle. In the triad, low food intake is what ultimately impairs reproductive and bone health. The female athlete triad is prevalent among athletes in sports that focus on thinness, weight class, endurance, or body image, such as ballet, figure skating, gymnastics, rowing, and running. Stress fractures, injuries, and nutritional deficiencies are extremely common in this population.

The best approach for the female athlete triad is early detection and prevention. The first aim of treatment is to increase your food intake and limit exercise energy expenditure to help restore the period and improve bone mineral density. Physical examinations are important to screen for signs and symptoms and helpful in detecting changes in weight, mood, fractures, injury, or a decline in athletic performance. Open lines of communication from athlete to coach are key.

The advice below is tailored mostly to secondary amenorrhea, hypothalamic amenorrhea, and the female athlete triad because they are all closely tied to one another. (See page 147.)

HOW DO I KNOW IF I HAVE AMENORRHEA?

There are no specific tests for this one, friends. This is a "diagnosis of exclusion," meaning clinicians rule out other conditions that could be interrupting the menstrual cycle. It's essential to get a physical exam and discuss your medical, menstrual, weight, and family history with your physician. You'll likely also get hormonal testing, a pelvic exam, and an ultrasound. By alleviating and treating potential underlying causes, it may help to reveal the true abnormality that's impacting your menstrual cycle.

NOTE: When detecting the cause of amenorrhea, remember that BMI and amenorrhea are not mutually exclusive. You can still have amenorrhea and be at a healthy BMI, and having a low BMI or being underweight doesn't always cause amenorrhea. You can still get your period at a low BMI and a high BMI. Dropping 10 pounds can stop menstruation so don't get caught up on BMI numbers, as it is not a direct measurement of health status. Because everyone's body is different (some require more energy while others require less), a friendly reminder not to compare yourself. Refocus on YOUR history and patterns of weight.

WHAT DO I DO NOW?

Although there isn't a magical cure-all, adopting new practices such as reducing stress, decreasing exercise, and eating more to nutritionally balance your diet (or putting on weight if you've recently lost weight) can help restore your period. It's not an exact science. No two bodies are 100% alike, but we do know these behavior modifications can make all the difference!

DISCLAIMER: I am a health care provider, but I am not your *personal* health care provider. My advice shouldn't stop you from seeing your own health care provider, getting a proper diagnosis, and following their recommendations for treatment.

MANAGING AMENORRHEA

INCREASE LOW LEPTIN

Fat is necessary to orchestrate your menstrual cycle. Leptin, a hormone derived from fat tissue, basically powers on your cycle by nudging reproductive hormones (FSH and LH) to get working. However, women with HA typically have low levels of leptin, especially if they intentionally remove fat from their diets. Leptin deficiency can result in the loss of a period because your body is no longer able to produce necessary reproductive hormones.

In fact, a raw food diet (defined as eating just fruits and vegetables) caused 70% of females to experience irregularities in their menstruation. This shows that the body needs more than just fruits and veggies to menstruate.[154] In research, when women reversed low leptin levels, it brought back their periods and increased ovulation by more than 50%.[155] After six months, an extra 360 calories/day resulted in a 3.5-pound weight gain, which restored menses and ovulation in women with exercise-related amenorrhea.[156] This proved that fat is essential to build hormones, prompt ovulation, and charge up the menstrual cycle.[157]

Therefore, boost leptin by increasing both your food and calorie intake. Pay more attention to eating more healthy fats at every meal and double or triple your regular serving size to build more leptin in the body. Eat more whole avocados, drizzle more olive oil to your meals, add grass-fed ghee or butter to your scrambled

---

154   https://www.ncbi.nlm.nih.gov/pubmed/10436305
155   https://www.ncbi.nlm.nih.gov/pubmed/21464293
156   https://www.ncbi.nlm.nih.gov/pubmed/25090245
157   https://www.ncbi.nlm.nih.gov/pubmed?term=10084564

eggs, snack on healthy nuts and seeds, and eat more frequently throughout the day.

INCREASE WEIGHT

Eating more and increasing weight (especially if you have a recent history of weight loss) is a powerful and effective strategy to treat HA. Women who recovered from HA showed an increase in their weight whereas non-recovered women showed a decrease or a weight that remained stable. Remember, although HA is common in women with a BMI of 20 or below, a significant weight loss (10 pounds or more) can trigger HA, even if the end weight is still considered to be in the "normal" or "overweight" BMI. It bears repeating, everyone is different so consider your own *weight history* as a factor in HA.

BODY MASS INDEX (BMI)	CLASSIFICATION
<18.5	Underweight
18.5-24.9	Normal weight
25-29.9	Overweight
>30.0	Obese

NOTE: To easily calculate your BMI, the CDC, NIH, and Mayo Clinic all have BMI calculators on their websites. Or, download an app like the BMI Calculator on your smartphone.

CUT BACK ON HIGH FIBER

A common characteristic among HA women is eating low-carb and high-fiber diets. Studies have found that women who adhered to high-fiber diets were more likely to have HA as well as low estrogen levels.[158] A possible explanation is that in HA, the body is fighting hard to increase estrogen. The body wants to find a happy medium of estrogen, not too much but not too little. Fiber acts like a broom

---

158   https://www.ncbi.nlm.nih.gov/pubmed?term=10084564

that sweeps estrogen out of the body, which can cause estrogen levels to dip too much. So, if you throw too much fiber into the equation, estrogen is unable to be restored back to adequate levels. That's no good!

In addition to estrogen, fiber was shown to also reduce LH and FSH, which can halt menstruation.[159] In studies, each 5 gram increase in fiber was linked to a significant association with an anovulatory cycle (where a woman doesn't release an egg), which can result in heavy bleeding in the next cycle and impaired fertility down the road.[160] Lower hormonal concentrations were also associated with higher fiber intakes, leading to more anovulatory cycles, which is a big risk factor for infertility.[161]

Fiber (both soluble and insoluble) keeps you full, which is generally a good thing, but in HA, it can suppress your appetite for too long and negatively impact your cycles. Until your cycle is restored, favor insoluble fiber over soluble fiber (see the food chart on page 157) and keep fiber intake below 20g per day.

AVOID SOY

In a systematic review and meta-analysis, isoflavones and soy protein (such as tofu, tempeh, edamame) didn't impact estrogen levels but did decrease FSH and LH in premenopausal women. A characteristic in HA is low levels of FSH and LH, which means eating isoflavones and soy could further reduce these vital hormones. To prevent FSH and LH from dipping even lower, a high intake of isoflavone-rich soy foods, such as soybeans, tofu, and edamame is not advisable.

---

159   https://www.ncbi.nlm.nih.gov/pubmed/19692496
160   https://www.ncbi.nlm.nih.gov/pubmed/19692496
161   https://www.ncbi.nlm.nih.gov/pubmed/19692496

BUILD BONES

Vitamin D keeps reproductive hormones in good condition and is essential to bone health as well. Maintaining good bone health is key in amenorrhea and in the female athlete triad. Low bone mineral density occurs in 22% to 50% of female athletes compared to 2% to 12% reported in the average population [162] If athletes are cutting out specific food groups (like dairy or fat) or undereating in general, they could be creating big nutritional gaps in their diet, such as low vitamin D and calcium. Osteopenia and osteoporosis, both conditions related to diminished bones, are long-term complications of amenorrhea and the female athlete triad. Plus, those with HA are more susceptible to weak bones and a compromise in bone health can up the odds for stress fractures or osteoporosis.[163, 164]

PROTECT YOUR HEART

Coronary artery disease (CAD) appears to be significantly associated with secondary amenorrhea. Women with exercise-related amenorrhea have a higher risk for elevated LDL, triglycerides, diabetes, and cholesterol than healthy women.[165] To safekeep your heart through food, aim for heart-healthy foods like whole grains, avocados, lentils, sweet potatoes, mushrooms, and olive oil, and antioxidant-rich foods such as walnuts and sunflower seeds. Balance your plate with proteins, healthy fats, and carbohydrates at every meal to prevent a blood sugar roller coaster.

162   https://www.ncbi.nlm.nih.gov/pmc/articles/PMC3435916/
163   https://www.ncbi.nlm.nih.gov/pmc/articles/PMC3435916/
164   https://www.ncbi.nlm.nih.gov/pubmed/2224267?dopt=Abstract
165   https://www.ncbi.nlm.nih.gov/pubmed/15572426/

EASE UP YOUR EXERCISE ROUTINE

It's time to take a break from the gym, ladies. Intense exercise has been associated with longer menstrual cycles, amenorrhea, and cycles without ovulation, whereas moderate exercise has more beneficial outcomes on health.[166] Vigorous training can psychologically contribute to higher anxiety and stress overload. The goal is to cut back from whatever physical activity you are doing, either completely or slightly, in order to restore your cycle. Athletes, work with your coach to come up with a realistic game plan to help you scale back on your physical activity without jeopardizing your career.

STRESS NO MORE

Stress can be a huge factor in the development of HA. In studies, the stress hormone cortisol was higher in women with low leptin, a common characteristic in both HA and the female athlete triad.[167] In fact, higher levels of cortisol were seen in amenorrhea exercisers versus regular menstruating exercisers.[168] Lowering stress is key because when measuring recovery of HA, lower cortisol was a common factor among those who no longer had HA.[169] Besides learning stress-reducing techniques such as meditation and deep breathing, foods with omega-3s, such as fish, nuts, and flaxseeds, have been shown to help lower depression, anxiety, and stress. Studies show that athletes may benefit from these types of foods the most.[170]

---

166   https://www.ncbi.nlm.nih.gov/pubmed/24173534
167   https://www.ncbi.nlm.nih.gov/pubmed?term=10084564
168   https://www.ncbi.nlm.nih.gov/pubmed/2267/1919
169   https://www.ncbi.nlm.nih.gov/pubmed/11836275
170   https://www.ncbi.nlm.nih.gov/pubmed/26836504

CONSIDER THERAPY

Disordered eating or eating disorders, often seen in the female athlete triad or HA, affects both the mind and the body. This psychological condition can often be accompanied by depression, anxiety, obsessive-compulsive disorder (OCD), low self-esteem, and a significant drive for thinness. In research, there was an increase in mortality rate among women with disordered eating, especially in those with anorexia nervosa.[171] HA patients reported higher depression, higher anxiety, and more sexual problems compared to healthy subjects.[172]

Overcoming denial and seeking help is the best place to start. Consider working with a psychotherapist or mental health professional (such as a psychologist, psychiatrist, clinical social worker, or licensed mental health counselor) who uses cognitive behavioral therapy (CBT) as part of their practice to uncover and address underlying emotional symptoms to improve quality of life. Cognitive behavioral therapy (CBT), a type of talk therapy that helps patients understand the thoughts and feelings that influence behavior and has been shown to be an effective treatment in those with HA. Find support groups and communities; your community could just be a #hashtag away. Search for #hypothalamicamenorrhea, #EDrecoveryispossible, #amenorrhearecovery on Twitter or Instagram. Two must-reads are *No Period. Now What?* by Nicola J. Rinaldi, PHD, and *Run Fast. Cook Fast. Eat Slow.* by Shalane Flanagan and Elyse Kopecky.

If you or someone you know wants to learn more about treatment options, contact the National Eating Disorder Association (NEDA)

---

171   https://www.ncbi.nlm.nih.gov/pubmed/21727255
172   https://www.ncbi.nlm.nih.gov/pubmed/26486482

(www.nationaleatingdisorders.org). The National Alliance on Mental Illness (NAMI) (www.nami.org) is also a good resource.

Soluble and Insoluble Fiber Food Examples

To help you distinguish the differences between soluble and insoluble fiber, I listed common foods and separated them according to their fiber makeup. Some foods have both soluble and insoluble fiber as indicated by the asterisk. Foods are not listed in any particular order.

FOODS	SOLUBLE FIBER EXAMPLES	INSOLUBLE FIBER EXAMPLES
Fruits	Apples	Apricots*
	Apricots*	Blueberries
	Avocado	Figs
	Bananas	Pear
	Blackberries	Raspberries
	Citrus fruits	Strawberries
	Kiwi	
	Prunes	
Vegetables	Artichokes	Beets
	Asparagus	Broccoli*
	Broccoli*	Brussels sprouts*
	Brussels sprouts*	Carrots*
	Cabbage	Corn
	Carrots*	Green beans
	Green peas	Kale, cooked
	Okra	Potato*
	Potato*	Squash
	Squash	Sweet potato*
	Sweet potato*	Tomato
	Zucchini	Turnip

FOODS	SOLUBLE FIBER EXAMPLES	INSOLUBLE FIBER EXAMPLES
Grains	Barley Brown rice Millet Oat bran Oatmeal* Popcorn Wheat bran* Wheat germ*	Oatmeal* Quinoa Wheat bran* Wheat germ*
Nuts	Brazil nuts Peanuts*	Almonds Peanuts* Walnuts
Seeds	Chia seeds Flaxseeds* Pumpkin seeds	Flaxseeds* Sesame seeds Sunflower seeds
Miscellaneous	Chicory Psyllium Tofu	
Legumes	Black beans Black-eyed peas Edamame Kidney beans* Navy beans Pinto beans White beans	Chickpeas Kidney beans* Lentils Lima beans Split peas

* Denotes both soluble and insoluble fiber

10

BOOST FERTILITY

What do all the other chapters (Polycystic Ovarian Syndrome, Amenorrhea, Thyroid Dysfunction, Endometriosis) have in common? You nailed it, they all deeply impact fertility. Whether you are trying to get pregnant or want to learn how to set up your body for fertility success down the road, this is the chapter for you! Optimal nutrition is critical for all women of childbearing age, even before starting a family. In fact, 1 out of 8 couples will have fertility issues so it's never too early to eat foods in favor of a more friendly reproductive environment.

A huge part of my nutrition practice focuses on how food can support women in their fertility journey. I've seen the success nutrition has on fertility; clients can make a few fundamental tweaks to their diet and lifestyle and get pregnant in the blink of an eye. In fact, diet and lifestyle adjustments have been shown to boost fertility by almost 70%.[173] That being said, I've also had clients who do everything right when it comes to their nutrition, and they are still unable to conceive naturally. Keep in mind that nutrition is just one piece of the complex fertility puzzle.

---

173   https://www.ncbi.nlm.nih.gov/pubmed/17978119

DISCLAIMER: If you follow these recommendations, it doesn't mean you will get pregnant, and if you don't follow my tips, it doesn't mean that you won't get pregnant. If fertility is on your mind, let's agree that eating better is a great place to start to stack the reproductive deck in your favor.

EAT FOR FERTILITY

Every cycle, the body continuously relies on the perfect cocktail of macro- and micronutrients that ultimately gives the A-OK for healthy embryo development and potential fertilization. Nutrients, such as zinc, vitamin D, and iron, have the power to turn on and off hormones and metabolic pathways in your reproductive system to nurture ovulation and a possible pregnancy.

Food holds the key to give the body the fertility green light. Each meal is an opportunity to get your nutritional ducks in a row to support fertility. One particular food won't get you pregnant overnight (and don't trust any companies that make these false promises!), but a smattering of nutrient-rich foods can positively tip the fertility scale in your direction. I will teach you which fertility-friendly nutrients to COPY + PASTE and which foods to CTRL-ALT-DELETE from your diet that could unknowingly be putting a wrench in your fertility. Without further ado...

EAT MORE FERTILITY-BOOSTING FOODS

Monounsaturated fat, omega-3 fatty acids, vegetables, iron from plants and supplements, low glycemic index foods, and full- or high-fat dairy were associated with a lower risk of ovulatory disorder infertility (see page 162).[174] Adherence to a healthy diet favoring mainly seafood, poultry, whole grains, fruits, and vegetables were linked to better fertility in women.[175] These dietary recommendations are quite similar to the Mediterranean diet, the number one diet in 2019 according to the *U.S. News and World Report*. If you want to learn more about the Mediterranean diet, see page 21.

Diet, Fertility, and Science

The largest and longest-running study to date followed the eating habits of over 18,000 nurses for eight years who did not have a history of infertility, as they tried to become pregnant or became pregnant. Prestigious researchers Drs. Jorge Chavarro and Walter Willett at the Harvard School of Public Health pooled together nutrition relationships and wrote the *The Fertility Diet* based on their findings. Last year, a literature review (a review's purpose is to summarize ALL the literature and research on nutrition and fertility and then offer dietary recommendations) conducted by Dr. Chavarro and colleagues further dissected the relationship between diet and fertility to help identify a few clear dietary patterns to promote fertility.[176] My dietary recommendations are based on these patterns and relationships (not to be confused with cause and effects), not from smaller, less extensive, or outdated studies.

174   https://www.ncbi.nlm.nlh.gov/pubmed/17978119
175   https://www.ncbi.nlm.nih.gov/pubmed/28844822
176   https://www.ncbi.nlm.nih.gov/pubmed/28844822

Recent research suggests that in those undergoing in vitro fertilization (IVF), a diet high in vitamin B12, vitamin D, dairy, soy, seafood rather than meat, low-pesticide produce, and folic acid supplements, proved to experience a more favorable outcome on fertility compared to when on the Mediterranean diet.[177]

What Is Ovulatory Disorder Infertility?

Ovulatory disorder infertility, also referred to as ovulatory infertility, is a leading cause of infertility. The process of ovulation, or releasing an egg, is either irregular or doesn't occur so pregnancy is unable to be achieved.

EAT MORE SEAFOOD

Up your seafood game. Women who eat eight servings or more of seafood per cycle have been shown to get pregnant sooner than those who rarely eat seafood.[178]

EAT MORE FULL- OR HIGH-FAT DAIRY

High-fat (or full-fat) dairy is the way to go. In studies, women who ate one or more servings of high-fat dairy foods per day were 27% less likely to be infertile.[179] Women who ate more low-fat dairy foods increased their risk of infertility, so simply said, swap your low-fat dairy with high-fat dairy to boost fertility.

177   https://www.ncbi.nlm.nih.gov/pubmed/30742825
178   https://academic.oup.com/jcem/advance-article-abstract/doi/10.1210/jc.2018-00385/5001729?redirectedFrom=fulltext
179   https://www.ncbi.nlm.nih.gov/pubmed/17978119

REDUCE YOUR RISKS

A high intake of saturated fat, red meat, trans fat, sugar, refined carbohydrates, soda, a BMI of less than 20, a BMI greater than 30, and physical inactivity were linked to lower fertility rates. FYI, it took women longer to get pregnant if they ate fast food four or more times per week compared to those who didn't eat any fast food.[180]

EAT MORE PLANTS

Factors such as stress, environmental pollutants, lack of sleep, excessive dieting, and excessive caffeine and alcohol consumption can deplete vitamins, minerals, and antioxidants needed to signal optimal fertility. Have no fear because eating more plants can help you recreate these nutrition-building blocks in your body. Plant-based proteins are the way to go for those trying to conceive. In studies, high protein intake from meat was linked to a 32% higher chance of developing ovulatory infertility.[181] Replacing animal sources of protein, especially red meat, with vegetable sources, such as nuts, seeds, green beans, and edamame, may reduce the risk of ovulatory infertility and protect against infertility.[182] By eating more vegetable proteins than animal proteins, the risk of ovulatory infertility can decrease by more than 50%.

Load up your next meal with plant-based proteins such as chickpeas, lentils, quinoa, and even artichokes. You can also get proteins through nuts and seeds such as Brazil nuts, sesame seeds, walnuts, and sunflower seeds. Not only do these foods check off the protein box, they also have nutrients to help improve egg quality such as zinc, magnesium, and selenium.

---

180   https://academic.oup.com/humrep/article/33/6/1063/4989162
181   https://www.ncbi.nlm.nih.gov/pubmed/17978119
182   https://www.ncbi.nlm.nih.gov/pubmed/18226626

Dark leafy greens and other nutrient-dense plant foods such as mushrooms, eggplant, kale, and cauliflower are also your friends. Think, the richer and deeper the color, the more nutritious! Vegetables like asparagus, broccoli, and kale also help deliver antioxidant MVP glutathione, which can increase egg quality. A good rule of thumb: half the food on your plate should always be veggies!

GET ENOUGH VITAMIN D

Vitamin D is like a stage mom. Just as a stage mom is heavily involved in her children's success, vitamin D is involved heavily in the success of the reproductive system. Vitamin D is very influential in achieving healthy egg development and can help power on reproductive hormones.[183] Vitamin D supplementation may also help improve IVF, making the chance for a successful procedure as much as four times higher.[184] Make sure to get enough vitamin D (both from food and as a supplement) as part of your daily routine.

FOLIC ACID + MYOINOSITOL

In PCOS patients, certain things work better together than by themselves, like Chip and Joanna Gaines from the popular reality show *Fixer Upper* on HGTV. The husband and wife duo showcase their individual strengths: Chip is the contractor who redesigns the framework of the house while Joanna is the interior designer. Joanna can decorate and work on floor plans, but without Chip, the house would still have outdated plumbing, electricity, and so on. Point is, it's better for them to team up to make the best result.

---

183   https://www.ncbi.nlm.nih.gov/pubmed/26035242
184   Ibid

Anyway, in PCOS patients, folic acid and myoinositol (see page 114) supplements work very well together as an effective treatment for promoting ovulation in women with fertility issues.[185, 186] Both supplements (2 x 2000mg myoinositol/day and 2 x 200mcg folic acid) have proven to be a safe and promising tool in restoring ovulation and managing symptoms and improvements in infertility for patients with PCOS. [187, 188]

INOSITOL: Referred to as vitamin B8, inositol is actually a naturally occurring sugar found in foods like buckwheat, beans, nuts, and citrus fruits. In research, two forms of inositol supplements are commonly used, myoinositol (MI) and D-chiro-inositol (DI). Inositol is found in food, whereas MI and DI are only found in supplements. Studies suggest these supplements may help to improve ovulation because they help sensitize cells to insulin and regulate insulin, which is necessary for ovulation.[189]

FOLATE: Also known as vitamin B9, folate helps to create new healthy red blood cells, DNA/RNA, and is instrumental in preventing birth defects like spina bifida, a neural tube defect. It's naturally found in foods; like oranges, eggs, beets, avocados, and asparagus.

FOLIC ACID: This is the synthetic form of folate used in vitamin supplements and in fortified food such as cereals, milk, and orange juice. It's advised to have sufficient amounts in the diet prior to conception; however, if the dietary intake is not adequate, it's recommended to take a prenatal vitamin containing 800mcg folic

185   https://www.ncbi.nlm.nih.gov/pubmed/25259724
186   https://www.hindawi.com/journals/ogi/2014/141020
187   https://www.ncbi.nlm.nih.gov/pubmed/29498933
188   https://www.ncbi.nlm.nih.gov/pmc/articles/PMC5011528
189   https://www.ncbi.nlm.nih.gov/pubmed/25259724

acid. This is because neural tube forms before many women know they are even pregnant.

SO...IS FAT GOOD FOR FERTILITY?

Unsaturated fats and omega-3 fatty acids (think walnuts, pumpkin seeds, flaxseeds, avocados) are essential to help boost fertility. These fats ignited hormones involved in ovulation. In fact, a study of 500 couples found that there was a shorter time getting pregnant in those that had more had more fat sources from lignans, such as flaxseed and sesame seeds, in their diet.[190]

A diet high in trans fats has been correlated to a greater risk of infertility and eating trans fats instead of carbohydrates increased fertility problems by 73%.[191] Thankfully, we can all breathe a sigh of relief because the FDA officially banned adding trans fats and partially hydrogenated oils (the primary source of artificial trans fats) to food in June 2018. However, the FDA has extended the deadline to January 2020 for some manufacturers to help transition their products into the marketplace. So just a friendly reminder to always read the label because partially hydrogenated oils can still be hiding in manufactured and packaged food products like baked goods, fried foods, and margarine.

Beyond trans fat, the more saturated fat intake in relation to monounsaturated or polyunsaturated fat intake, the greater the risk for ovulation issues.[192] Time to make room for more chia seeds, hemp seeds, pumpkin seeds, and healthy unsaturated oils like walnut, avocado, olive, or flaxseed oil in your pantry?

---

190   https://academic.oup.com/jn/article/144/3/352/4615608
191   https://www.ncbi.nlm.nih.gov/pubmed/17209201
192   https://www.ncbi.nlm.nih.gov/pubmed/18226626

GET YOUR IRON

Beans, lentils, spinach, oh my! It's a good idea to fill up on iron-rich plant-based foods to boost fertility. A diet rich in iron, especially coming from plants such as quinoa, cashews, and pumpkin seeds, can lower the risk of ovulatory infertility.[193] Plus, iron supplementation in conjunction with iron-rich plant proteins can reduce reproductive disorders like ovulatory infertility by 40%.[194] This year the *Journal of Nutrition* found that heme iron, coming from meat, has no effect on how long it takes a woman to conceive. Nonheme iron, found in vegetables and in supplements, did slightly increase the chance of pregnancy only for women who were more likely to be iron deficient due to heavy menses, had short menstrual cycles, or had previously given birth.

So next time you are building your plate, make sure to get a healthy serving of nonheme iron-rich foods like edamame, chickpeas, and peas, and don't forget to take your iron supplements, especially if you are deficient!

DON'T FORGET MULTIVITAMINS

Women who took multivitamins every day had a 41% lower chance of infertility. Vitamins that had adequate B vitamins (particularly B12 and folic acid), iron, and omega-3 have been shown to have positive effects on fertility and decreased the risk of ovulatory infertility.[195, 196] It's still important to cast a wide nutritional net with your diet so you don't miss out on key fertility nutrients like zinc and vitamin D. High-quality foods are more important than high-quality vitamins so if you don't want to splurge to get the organic,

---

193   https://www.ncbi.nlm.nih.gov/pubmed/17077236
194   https://www.ncbi.nlm.nih.gov/pubmed/17624345
195   Ibid
196   https://www.ncbi.nlm.nih.gov/pubmed/28844822

pricey, and premium vitamin brand, don't sweat. Choose a vitamin that's easy to find, digests well in your belly, won't burn a hole in your wallet and, most importantly, you remember to take every day! According to research, 20% of ovulatory infertility may be avoided if women consume three or more multivitamins per week, so don't forget it, girlfriend! [197]

Vitamin C + Iron

You've probably remember from other chapters, but it's worth repeating. Plant-based sources of iron (known as nonheme) are stubborn and difficult for your body to absorb. At your next meal, add some vitamin C to your plant-based proteins (such as a squeeze of Meyer lemon, blistered peppers, charred broccoli, or a puffy sweet potato) to help your body break down and enhance the absorption of nonheme iron. Trust me, your body will say yum + THANK YOU at the same time.

EMBRACE SOY

No need to fear soy! Researchers found that eating soy was not related to poor fertility. In fact, higher intakes of soy and soy supplements appear to have beneficial effects among women undergoing infertility treatments.[198, 199]

197   https://www.ncbi.nlm.nih.gov/pubmed/17624345
198   https://www.ncbi.nlm.nih.gov/pubmed/28844822
199   https://www.ncbi.nlm.nih.gov/pubmed/30742825

FLUID EFFECTS

COFFEE + CAFFEINE

No need to ditch your coffee either! In studies, coffee drinkers weren't any more or less likely to have trouble getting pregnant than women who didn't drink coffee.[200] Even in couples undergoing infertility treatment with assisted reproductive technologies (ART), the latest research from July 2019 found no effect from coffee on fertility success.[201] And research suggests that caffeine in general can be consumed in moderation without negatively impacting fertility.[202] In fact, caffeine consumption has been linked to a lower frequency of random ovulation and a lower risk of infertility due to a lack of ovulation among healthy women.[203] So don't worry ladies, you can still sip your caffeinated green tea and espresso, and love your matcha latte–a latte!

ALCOHOL

Yes, prior to pregnancy, it is OK to drink alcohol in moderation! One drink per day does not negatively impact fertility. Plus, infertility is not any more common in those who have one drink per day than those who do not drink at all. This may be surprising but the specific type of alcohol doesn't hinder fertility rates, whether it is wine, beer, or spirits.[204] Alcohol, just like caffeine, has little effect, good or bad, on fertility.[205]

200   https://www.ncbi.nlm.nih.gov/pubmed/17978119
201   https://www.ncbi.nlm.nih.gov/pubmed/31043232
202   https://www.ncbi.nlm.nih.gov/pubmed/28844822
203   https://www.ncbi.nlm.nih.gov/pubmed/31043232
204   https://www.ncbi.nlm.nih.gov/pubmed/17978119
205   https://www.ncbi.nlm.nih.gov/pubmed/28844822

SODA

In research, while coffee, diet soda, tea, juice, and alcohol didn't seem to affect fertility, women drinking two or more caffeinated sodas a day were 50% more likely to have ovulatory infertility than women who drank less than one caffeinated soda per week.[206] Recent studies also suggest that the consumption of sugar-sweetened beverages (especially sodas and energy drinks) are linked to lower fertility rates.[207]

ORGANIC PRODUCE IS BEST

To keep exposure to hormone and endocrine disruptors, like pesticides, to a minimum, eat organic produce when possible. Eating more low-pesticide-residue produce in comparison to high-pesticide-residue produce was shown to have more favorable outcomes in women undergoing IVF.[208] You want those nutritious fruits and veggies to work with your hormones, not interfere with them!

The Environmental Working Group (EWG), a nonprofit organization dedicated to protecting human health and the environment, creates the annual "Dirty Dozen" and "Clean Fifteen" list to show consumers the fruits and veggies they should buy organic when possible. The "Dirty Dozen" is listed from dirtiest to least dirty where "Clean Fifteen" is listed from cleanest to least clean (see page 129).

---

206   https://www.ncbi.nlm.nih.gov/pubmed/17978119
207   https://journals.lww.com/epidem/Abstract/2018/05000/Intake_of_Sugar_sweetened_Beverages_and.8.aspx
208   https://www.ncbi.nlm.nih.gov/pubmed/30742825

KITCHEN TIPS

- **AVOID BPA AS MUCH AS POSSIBLE.** A harmful chemical found in plastic water bottles, food storage containers, and some canned foods, BPA can be a hormone disruptor. Look for BPA-free products, avoid eating or drinking from products with recycling symbols No. 3 or No. 7, and get refillable water bottles. I love the water bottle companies Healthy Human, BKR, Swell, and Welly.

- **GO TO A LOCAL FARMER'S MARKET** for less-expensive, seasonal organic produce and to support your local farmers, agriculture, and economy.

- **COOK FOODS AT LOWER TEMPERATURES.** Cooking food at high temperatures increases its susceptibility of developing inflammatory compounds such as advanced glycation end products (AGEs). AGEs tend to accumulate in the body and have been linked to PCOS-related infertility, ovulatory dysfunction, and insulin resistance.[209, 210] Reduce exposure to AGEs by grilling less, cooking foods at lower temperatures, and marinating proteins beforehand in an acid like lemon juice, lime juice, or vinegar. If you need to cook at high temperatures, use cooking oils that can withstand high heat temperatures such as coconut, grapeseed, and avocado oil, and use sparingly.

MAINTAIN A HEALTHY WEIGHT

Many cases of infertility can be traced to weight issues. According to the American Society for Reproductive Medicine (ASRM), more

209   https://www.ncbi.nlm.nih.gov/pubmed/26690206
210   https://www.ncbi.nlm.nih.gov/pubmed/24173721

than 70% of women who have weight-related infertility could get pregnant without fertility treatments if they bring their weight to a healthier level. Researchers found a higher risk of ovulatory infertility in those with a BMI below 20 or above 24, so it's important to find a happy medium.[211] Both overweight and underweight women pose the risk of having hormonal imbalances that negatively impact the cycle and can ultimately affect the quality of her eggs. In studies, losing or gaining weight to achieve a normal BMI not only increased pregnancy rates but also decreased pregnancy complications.[212]

Be Your Own Detective

If your weight won't budge, look under the hood as to why weight loss or weight gain is difficult and ask your doctor to rule out PCOS, thyroid issues, and endometriosis, and double-check your hormone panels. Be sure to bring up stress levels, sleep, work/life balance, and family or relationship issues. These conditions could be impacting your weight as well as your fertility status.

DISCLAIMER: I've discussed that the BMI may not be the best measure of overall health. However, researchers use the BMI as a way to categorize participants in their studies. To better grasp an understanding of your own picture of health beyond the BMI classification, I encourage you to assess muscle mass, body fat, genetics, and family weight history.

211   https://www.ncbi.nlm.nih.gov/pubmed/11880759
212   https://www.ncbi.nlm.nih.gov/pubmed/17978119

OVERWEIGHT

Overweight or obese women have more leptin, which are fat cells that store sex hormones. So, the more fat cells, the more sex hormones. Therefore, you may be more likely to have imbalances in insulin, estrogen, testosterone, and FSH and LSH, which are the forces behind proper egg development and a successful ovulation.

Obesity is a significant cause of anovulatory infertility. Among obese women, the infertility rate was shown to increase by 4% for every additional BMI unit.[213] Less frequent menstruation and cycles without ovulation are more common in overweight and obese women.[214]

UNDERWEIGHT

A BMI below normal may also prevent ovulation and a healthy cycle. Plus, low leptin can negatively impact hormone production, which may prevent ovulation. (See Chapter 9, Amenorrhea for a more in-depth discussion). Eating more fat and gaining weight may help trigger ovulation, enhance fertility, and adequately prepare the body for a healthy pregnancy.[215]

Overweight women who lose 5% to 10% of their body weight and underweight women who gain a few pounds can dramatically improve their chances of conception. The good news is that small steps in the right direction can make a big difference to improve your chances of getting pregnant.

213   https://www.ncbi.nlm.nih.gov/pubmed/19828554
214   https://www.ncbi.nlm.nih.gov/pubmed/17978119
215   https://www.ncbi.nlm.nih.gov/pmc/articles/PMC3943486

TRACY'S TOP FERTILITY-FOCUSED GUIDELINES

1. Eat less trans fats, less saturated fat, and more mono- and polyunsaturated fats such as cashews, olives, peanut butter, pecans, hazelnuts, avocados.

2. Combine ovulation-enhancing unsaturated fats, such as olive oil, pine nuts, and almonds with slow-digesting carbohydrates such as wild rice, brown rice, wheat berries, and lentils.

3. Incorporate plant-based proteins at every meal, such as nuts, seeds, green peas, lentils, and beans.

4. Eat eight or more seafood servings per month, with a focus on omega-3-rich fish, such as salmon, trout, and sardines.

5. Arm yourself with more omega-3-rich foods like walnuts, omega-3-fortified eggs, chia seeds, and flaxseeds.

6. Swap out skim and low-fat dairy foods with full-fat dairy every day. Yes, that means real cheese and whole milk!

7. Eat organic and grass-fed red meat once or twice per week.

8. Swap refined starches and potatoes for bean-based pasta and whole grain carbohydrates such as farro, oats, and brown rice.

9. Eat 5 cups of vegetables and 3 cups of fruits per day, especially those rich in vitamins A, C, and E, to help deliver antioxidants.

10. Eat more foods full of iron and folate, such as spinach, lentils, sweet potatoes, and oranges.

11. Consume tea, coffee, soy, and alcohol in moderation.

12. Get at least seven to eight hours of sleep each night.

13. Get your BMI to a healthy range.

14. If you smoke, stop!

15. Exercise, choosing a moderate/vigorous activity at least four days/week for 30 to 60 minutes.

16. Take a multivitamin with iron, folic acid, vitamin D, calcium, and omega-3 fatty acids.

Vitamin + Mineral Fertility Nutrition Checklist

VITAMIN/MINERAL	AMOUNT	BEST SOURCES
Calcium *Calcium carbonate is recommended form* *Multivitamin may not have calcium, may have to take as a separate supplement*	1,000 mg	Spinach, black eyed peas, ready-to-eat cereals, collard greens, sardines, soybeans, white beans, fresh or canned salmon, kale, tofu, baked beans
Vitamin D *Vitamin D3, cholecalciferol, is recommended form* *Take as an additional separate supplement, standard multivitamin only contains ~400IU vitamin D*	1,000IU	Fortified breakfast cereals, egg yolk, milk, cheese, yogurt, mushrooms, salmon, fortified alternative milk (almond, soy, oat, cashew)
Iron *Ferrous sulfate is recommended form* *Take as an additional separate supplement, standard multivitamin contains <40mg iron* *Favor nonheme sources over heme sources*	40 to 80mg	Nonheme: Fortified breakfast cereal, pumpkin seeds, soybeans, spinach (cooked), red kidney beans (cooked), lima beans (cooked), cashews (roasted), enriched rice (cooked), dried fruit Heme: Red meat, poultry, fish

VITAMIN/MINERAL	AMOUNT	BEST SOURCES
Folic acid *L-methylfolate aka 5-MTHF is recommended form* *Take as an additional separate supplement, standard multivitamin typically has 400mcg to prevent neural tube defects but studies show benefits of increasing the recommendation to improve ovulation + conception*	700 to 800mcg	Fortified breakfast cereals, white rice, lentils (cooked), pasta, garbanzo beans, spinach (cooked), citrus, asparagus (cooked), pita bread, orange juice
Coenzyme Q10 *An antioxidant that can protect the reproductive system*	400mg	Fatty fish like salmon, herring, sardines, and mackerel, spinach, strawberries, organ meats, pork, beef, chicken
Omega-3 Fatty Acids *DHA and EPA are recommended absorbable forms*	1200mg	Flaxseeds, omega-3-enriched eggs, salmon, trout, sardines, walnuts
Multivitamin	Get a prenatal version when possible (even before you get pregnant!)	SmartyPants New Chapter Pure Synergy Rainbow Light Garden of Life Mama Bird Thorne HUM Olly Nordic Naturals

Source: https://www.ncbi.nlm.nih.gov/pubmed/17624345, https://www.ncbi.nlm.nih.gov/pubmed/28844822

RECIPES

Now that you've come this far, you must be starving...let's eat! I've compiled a ton of recipes (breakfast, lunch, dinner, snacks, and desserts) that are in favor of a healthier menstrual cycle. No matter the day of the cycle, the ingredients in the recipe are specifically tailored to provide your body with synergistic nutrients to balance hormones, boost energy, and ensure that you become a menstrual maven! To help those who are food cycling, I've called out the phase (menstrual, follicular, ovulatory, luteal/PMS) of your cycle that the recipe will best support. Note that PMS can happen in the beginning of the menstrual phase or toward the tail end of the luteal phase, so use the PMS-tagged recipes whenever it may strike!

I've flagged recipes that are gluten-free, dairy-free, and vegetarian to help you stick to these nutritional guidelines. If the recipe can be modified toward gluten-free, dairy-free, or vegetarian, I've included alternative options in the ingredients list. I'm a sucker for easy leftovers so if the serving size says 2, have 1 serving now and save the other for later (or freeze the rest). Also, I love eating breakfast for dinner so if you feel so inclined to change up the rules, I fully support you! Now, let's eat our way to a better period, one bite at a time. And that's the story here, ladies–period!

SAMPLE MEAL PLAN

Menstrual Phase Sample Meal Plan

	BREAKFAST	LUNCH	DINNER	SNACK
Day 1	Strawberries 'n' Dream Overnight Oats (page 193)	Easy Slow Cooker Lentil Soup (page 253) + 1 slice Ezekiel bread with ½ avocado	Loaded Spaghetti Squash Boats (page 235)	1 small orange + ¼ cup Roasted Rosemary Walnuts (page 207)
Day 2	Eggs and Coconutty Vegetables (page 188) + ½ grapefruit	Loaded Spaghetti Squash Boats (page 235)	Chicken and Strawberry Fields for Dinner (page 246)	2 Pretty Pretty Chocolate Pumpkin Morning Muffins (page 210)
Day 3	Pumpkin Patch Overnight Oats (page 184)	Chicken and Strawberry Fields for Dinner (page 246)	Bok Choy and Tofu (page 223)	1 cup sliced yellow or red peppers + 2 tablespoons Sweet Pea Hummus (page 212)
Day 4	Turmeric Avocado Toast with Sprouted Ezekiel Bread (page 198)	Bok Choy and Tofu (page 223)	Butternut Squash and Kale Frittata (page 237)	8 strawberries + ¼ cup Honey Turmeric Nuts (page 206)
Day 5	Wild Blueberry Overnight Oats (page 197)	Butternut Squash and Kale Frittata (page 237)	Pumpkin Pesto Pasta (page 239)	1 small grapefruit + ¼ cup Honey Turmeric Nuts (page 206)
Day 6	Strawberries 'n' Dream Overnight Oats (page 193)	Easy Slow Cooker Lentil Soup (page 253) + 1 slice Ezekiel bread with 2 tablespoons hummus	Chicken and Strawberry Fields for Dinner (page 246)	1 small orange + ¼ cup Rosemary Roasted Walnuts (page 207)
Day 7	Turmeric Avocado Toast with Sprouted Ezekiel Bread (page 198)	Loaded Spaghetti Squash Boats (page 235)	Butternut Squash and Kale Frittata (page 237)	2 Pretty Pretty Chocolate Pumpkin Morning Muffins (page 210)

Follicular Phase Sample Meal Plan

	BREAKFAST	LUNCH	DINNER	SNACK
Day 1	Cereal Delight (page 186)	Coconut-Infused Butternut Squash Soup (page 219)	Parm Cheese and Broccoli Pasta (page 216)	1 piece Gluten-Free Pumpkin Bread (page 213) with 1 teaspoon butter or ghee
Day 2	Morning Mint Berry Chia Pudding (page 191)	Parm Cheese and Broccoli Pasta (page 216)	Sweet Potato Tacos (page 240)	1 small orange + ¼ cup Roasted Rosemary Walnuts (page 207)
Day 3	Cinnamon Sweet Potato Yogurt Bowl (page 199)	Edamame Pesto and Goat Cheese Toast (page 232)	Rotisserie Chicken Detox Salad (page 238)	Tropical Green Smoothie (page 209)
Day 4	Sweet (Berry) Dreams Chia Pudding (page 187)	Rotisserie Chicken Detox Salad (page 238)	Loaded Spaghetti Squash Bouls (page 235)	1 cup sugar snap peas + 2 tablespoons Sweet Pea Hummus (page 212)
Day 5	Cereal Delight (page 186)	Edamame Pesto and Goat Cheese Toast (page 232)	Parm Cheese and Broccoli Pasta (page 216)	1 piece Gluten-Free Pumpkin Bread (page 213) with 1 teaspoon butter or ghee
Day 6	Cinnamon Sweet Potato Yogurt Bowl (page 199)	Coconut-Infused Butternut Squash Soup (page 219)	Sweet Potato Tacos (page 240)	Tropical Green Smoothie (page 209)

Ovulatory Phase Sample Meal Plan

	BREAKFAST	LUNCH	DINNER	SNACK
Day 1	Chunky Monkey Chia Seed Pudding (page 195)	Sweet Potato Avocado Rice Bowl (page 221)	Creamy Roasted Garlic and Cauliflower Soup (page 217) + Smashed Potatoes with Garlic Pumpkin Seed Pesto (page 228)	1 cup carrots, 2 tablespoons Sweet Pea Hummus (page 212)
Day 2	Avocado Quinoa Bregg-fast Bowl (page 185)	Pineapple Cauliflower Fried Rice (page 233)	Easy Slow Cooker Lentil Soup (page 253) + Maple Seed Butter-Glazed Carrots (page 214)	3 Spirulina Energy Balls (page 202)
Day 3	Blueberry Carrot Cake Overnight Oats (page 189)	Easy Slow Cooker Lentil Soup (page 253) + Maple Seed Butter-Glazed Carrots (page 214)	Cauliflower Grits (page 249) served over 2 cups spinach	1 apple, 2 tablespoons nut butter, dash of cinnamon

Luteal Phase Sample Meal Plan

	BREAKFAST	LUNCH	DINNER	SNACK
Day 1	Eggs and Coconutty Vegetables (page 188) + 1 banana	Peaches and Cream Toast (page 220)	Loaded Baked Sweet Potato with Beans (page 244)	3 to 4 Apricot and Sunflower Energy Bites (page 203)
Day 2	Chunky Monkey Chia Seed Pudding (page 195)	Loaded Baked Sweet Potato with Beans (page 244)	Moroccan Quinoa Salad (page 226)	1 string cheese + 1 apple
Day 3	Vanilla-Spiced Date Caramel Sauce and Vanilla Yogurt (page 201)	Eggocado Open-Faced Sandy (page 225)	Quinoa-Stuffed Acorn Squash (page 241)	3 to 4 Apricot and Sunflower Energy Bites (page 203)
Day 4	Strawberries 'n' Dream Overnight Oats (page 193)	Quinoa-Stuffed Acorn Squash (page 241)	Black Bean Quinoa Burgers (page 242) + Maple Seed Butter Glazed Carrots	49 pistachios + 20 grapes
Day 5	No-Bake P.B.O. Energy Squares (page 196), 1 cup Greek yogurt, 1 cup blueberries	Black Bean Quinoa Burgers (page 242) + Maple Seed Butter-Glazed Carrots (page 214)	Easy Slow Cooker Lentil Soup (page 253) + Side of 1 cup roasted broccoli with lemon	1 cup Crispy Chickpeas (page 205) + 1 cup carrots
Day 6	PB Chocolate Oat Milk Overnight Oats (page 194)	Vegetarian Quinoa Bowl with Kale and Roasted Vegetables (page 247)	Loaded Spaghetti Squash Boats (page 235)	Choco-nutty Monkey Smoothie (page 211)
Day 7	Chocolate Banana Bread Chia Pudding (page 190)	Loaded Spaghetti Squash Boats (page 235)	Salmon and Shredded Brussels Sprout Tacos (page 251)	¼ cup Honey Turmeric Nuts (page 206) + ½ grapefruit

PMS Sample Meal Plan

	BREAKFAST	LUNCH	DINNER	SNACK
Day 1	PB Chocolate Oat Milk Overnight Oats (page 194)	Tahini, Kale, and Farro Stuffed Sweet Potato (page 230)	Loaded Spaghetti Squash Boats (page 235)	Choco-nutty Smoothie (page 211)
Day 2	Morning Honey Lemon Quinoa Parfait (page 200)	Cauliflower Grits (page 249) over 2 cups spinach	Vegetarian Quinoa Bowl with Kale and Roasted Vegetables (page 247)	¼ cup walnuts + 1 cup blackberries
Day 3	Golden Milk Overnight Oats (page 192)	Vegetarian Quinoa Bowl with Kale and Roasted Vegetables (page 247)	Salmon and Shredded Brussels Sprout Tacos (page 251)	1 piece Gluten-Free Peanut Butter Banana Bread (page 204) + 2 tablespoons nut butter
Day 4	Chocolate Banana Bread Chia Pudding (page 190)	Salmon and Shredded Brussels Sprout Tacos (page 251)	Pineapple Cauliflower Fried Rice (page 233)	Chocolate Zucchini Smoothie (page 208)
Day 5	Cinnamon Apple Pie Overnight Oats (page 186)	Loaded Baked Sweet Potato with Beans (page 244)	Quinoa-Stuffed Acorn Squash (page 241)	¼ cup Honey Turmeric Nuts (page 206) + ½ grapefruit

Dessert options for all phases:

- 3 Date and Peanut Butter Frozen Bites (page 260)
- Clementines and Dark Chocolate Fudge Sauce (page 263)
- 2 or 3 Dark Chocolate Peanut Butter Cups (page 261)
- Dark Chocolate and Cranberry Fudge Bars (page 258)
- 1 square of Pumpkin Spice Blondies (page 257)

BREAKFAST

Pumpkin Patch Overnight Oats

Who doesn't want to start off their menstrual cycle with satisfying and heart-healthy oats? Not only will the heart-warming nutmeg soothe cramps and inflammation, but the pumpkin seeds will provide a much-needed dose of zinc, a mineral that you can become deficient in during your period. And don't forget, zinc is key to proper egg follicle development. A big thank you to pumpkin seeds for delivering these helpful nutritional properties to our bodies!

SERVING SIZE: 1   **TOTAL TIME:** 5 minutes to prep, refrigerate overnight

Gluten-free, Dairy-free, Vegetarian

½ cup rolled oats

1 cup soy milk or milk of choice

1 teaspoon pumpkin pie spice

½ teaspoon ground cinnamon

¼ teaspoon ground nutmeg

2 tablespoons pumpkin seeds

½ Bartlett pear, chopped

1. Combine the oats with your milk of choice in a mason jar.

2. Add the pumpkin pie spice, cinnamon, nutmeg, pumpkin seeds, and chopped pear to the mason jar, and mix ingredients together.

3. Seal with a lid and refrigerate overnight.

4. Enjoy the next morning either at home or on the go. Serve cold.

Avocado Quinoa Bregg-fast Bowl

This bregg-fast bowl is nothing short of delicious and nutritious. During ovulation, you may not have the biggest appetite and may be inclined to skimp out on a well-balanced diet. That's why this bowl is packed with key nutrients from the avocado, egg, and quinoa, all of which will ensure you are hitting your macronutrients while still feeling light on your toes and ready to tackle the day!

SERVING SIZE: 1   **TOTAL TIME:** 45 minutes

Gluten-free, Dairy-free, Vegetarian

¼ cup quinoa

2 teaspoons olive oil, divided

1 cup halved and quartered Brussels sprouts

1 egg

1 cup fresh arugula

1 tablespoon pumpkin seeds

½ avocado, sliced

1 tablespoon tahini

1 teaspoon sesame seeds

Himalayan salt and pepper

1. Cook the quinoa according to package instructions and set aside.

2. Meanwhile, heat 1 teaspoon of olive oil in small, nonstick pan for 1 minute on medium heat, and then add the Brussels sprouts. Sauté for 15 minutes or until tender.

3. Using another small, nonstick pan, heat the remaining olive oil on medium heat. After 1 minute, crack the egg into the center of the pan and fry until the white has set, roughly 5 minutes.

4. In a large salad bowl, mix together the arugula, cooked quinoa, cooked Brussels sprouts, and pumpkin seeds. Place the sliced avocado and the fried egg on top of the salad.

5. Drizzle with tahini and sprinkle sesame seeds on top. Season with Himalayan salt and pepper to taste before serving.

Cereal Delight

SERVING SIZE: 1   **TOTAL TIME:** 3 minutes

Dairy-free, Vegetarian

¾ cup of your favorite cereal (Vans, Cascadian Farm Organic, Nature's Path)

½ cup fresh blueberries

2 tablespoons chopped walnuts

1 cup soy milk or milk of choice

1 tablespoon ground flaxseeds

1. Add the cereal, blueberries, and walnuts to a cereal bowl.

2. Pour the soy milk over the cereal and sprinkle flaxseeds on top.

Cinnamon Apple Pie Overnight Oats

SERVING SIZE: 1   **TOTAL TIME:** 5 minutes to prep, refrigerate overnight

Gluten-free, Dairy-free, Vegetarian

¼ cup rolled oats

½ cup walnut milk

2 tablespoons chopped walnuts

1 Granny Smith apple, chopped

1 teaspoon ground cinnamon

1. Combine the oats with the walnut milk in a mason jar.

2. Add the walnuts, chopped apple, and cinnamon to the mason jar, and mix the ingredients together.

3. Seal with a lid and refrigerate overnight.

4. Enjoy the next morning either at home or on the go. Serve cold and top with more cinnamon, if desired.

Sweet (Berry) Dreams Chia Pudding

Sweet dreams are made of...chia seeds! Chia seeds are overflowing with fiber, a key nutrient in the follicular phase that fights for hormonal balance. The fiber in the chia seeds keep estrogen at optimum levels, which is key in helping ward off PMS. Plus, the frozen blueberries are a secret weapon in this breakfast, providing powerful antioxidants to the body and helping to protect the developing follicle that's ready to be released in the upcoming ovulatory phase.

SERVING SIZE: 1   **TOTAL TIME:** 5 minutes to prep, refrigerate overnight

Gluten-free, Dairy-free, Vegetarian

¾ cup almond milk or milk of choice

3 tablespoons chia seeds

1 teaspoon vanilla extract

1 teaspoon honey

½ cup frozen blueberries

1 teaspoon ground cinnamon

1 tablespoon pumpkin seeds

1. Combine your milk of choice with the chia seeds in a mason jar.

2. Add the vanilla extract, honey, frozen blueberries, cinnamon, and pumpkin seeds to the mason jar, and mix the ingredients together.

3. Seal with a lid and refrigerate overnight.

4. Enjoy the next morning either at home or on the go. Serve cold, and top with more cinnamon, if desired.

Eggs and Coconutty Vegetables

This dynamic duo of eggs and veggies will set your body up for major cycle success. The veggies (like spinach, cauliflower, broccoli) are key to keeping your liver in tip-top shape while maintaining perfect hormonal balance. Eggs deliver an abundance of fat-soluble vitamins like A, D, E, and K, all which help to build a strong and healthy endometrial lining in the uterus to either support a pregnancy or to be shed during the next period. That's why this dish works well in both the menstrual and luteal phase.

SERVING SIZE: 2   **TOTAL TIME:** 7 minutes

Gluten-free, Dairy-free, Vegetarian

1 teaspoon cold-pressed coconut oil

1 cup frozen vegetable mix (carrots, cauliflower, broccoli, green beans)

1 cup raw spinach

½ teaspoon ground turmeric

pinch of sea salt

pinch of pepper

2 (omega-3–enriched) eggs, whisked

1 tablespoon sesame seeds or flaxseeds, depending on the day of cycle

1. Add the coconut oil to a small frying pan over medium heat.

2. After 1 minute, add the frozen vegetables. Let them thaw for 2 to 3 minutes in the pan.

3. Add the spinach, turmeric, salt, and pepper, and sauté for 1 minute.

4. Add the whisked eggs and scramble with a wooden spoon, about 2 to 3 minutes.

5. Top with your choice of seeds, adding more salt, pepper, and turmeric, if desired.

Blueberry Carrot Cake Overnight Oats

Carrot cake for breakfast? You better believe that this breakfast recipe will transport you from breakfast to dessert in a moment's notice! *Bonus Tip*: During ovulation, you may be craving more time in the bedroom rather than in the kitchen, so this breakfast is superfast and easy to make the night before. That way, you'll have more energy to get down to business (if you know what I mean!).

SERVING SIZE: 1 **TOTAL TIME:** 10 minutes to prep, refrigerate overnight

Gluten-free, Vegetarian

¼ cup finely grated carrots

¼ cup nonfat vanilla Greek yogurt or dairy-free yogurt

½ oup unsweetened almond milk

¼ cup rolled oats

¼ cup frozen or fresh blueberries

½ teaspoon ground cinnamon

2 tablespoons chopped walnuts

1. Add the carrots, yogurt, milk, oats, blueberries, cinnamon, and walnuts to a mason jar and mix the ingredients together.

2. Seal with a lid and refrigerate overnight.

3. Enjoy the next morning either at home or on the go. Serve cold, topped with more cinnamon, if desired.

Chocolate Banana Bread Chia Pudding

SERVING SIZE: 1   **TOTAL TIME:** 5 minutes to prep, refrigerate overnight

Gluten-free, Dairy-free, Vegetarian

¾ cup almond milk
or milk of choice

3 tablespoons chia seeds

1 tablespoon cacao nibs

1 teaspoon ground cinnamon

½ banana, mashed

1. Combine your milk of choice with the chia seeds in a mason jar.

2. Add the cacao nibs and cinnamon, and top with the mashed banana, then mix the ingredients together.

3. Seal with a lid and refrigerate overnight.

4. Enjoy the next morning either at home or on the go. Serve cold, topped with more cinnamon, if desired.

Morning Mint Berry Chia Pudding

This bright flavor combo is the answer that your taste buds are looking for this morning. The undeniable antioxidants spewing from the raspberries and goji berries will help repair any tissues that may have been inflamed during the menstrual phase. Soy milk will ensure the delivery of phytoestrogens, helping to keep estrogen levels in check. Plus, mint offers calming effects, which can also heal the body after you've had your period. And did I mention that mint may even help you tackle those stressful morning spreadsheets without wanting to pull your hair out? Sign me up!

SERVING SIZE: 1   **TOTAL TIME:** 5 minutes to prep, refrigerate overnight

Gluten-free, Dairy-free, Vegetarian

¾ cup soy milk or milk of choice

3 tablespoons chia seeds

2 tablespoons dried goji berries

1 tablespoon chopped fresh mint

¼ cup fresh or frozen raspberries

1. Combine your milk of choice with the chia seeds in a mason jar.

2. Add the goji berries, mint, and raspberries, and mix the ingredients together.

3. Seal with a lid and refrigerate overnight.

4. Enjoy the next morning either at home or on the go. Serve cold.

Golden Milk Overnight Oats

My fave PMS breakfast helps you go from zero to hero in no time. I'd be lying if I said I didn't eat this breakfast straight for 1 week leading up to my period, it's just that good! The healing properties of turmeric will soothe your uterus as it starts to wind up for your period. Plus, your taste buds will be appeased (without feeling overkill) by the natural sugars in the agave and coconut milk.

SERVING SIZE: 1   **TOTAL TIME:** 5 minutes to prep, refrigerate overnight

Gluten-free, Dairy-free, Vegetarian

1 cup coconut milk or milk of choice

½ cup rolled oats

1 teaspoon chia seeds

¼ teaspoon ground turmeric

1 tablespoon agave

⅛ teaspoon ground cinnamon

pinch of pepper

pinch of Himalayan salt

1. Combine your milk of choice with the oats in a mason jar.

2. Add the chia seeds, ground turmeric, agave, cinnamon, pepper, and salt, and mix the ingredients together.

3. Seal with a lid and refrigerate overnight.

4. Enjoy the next morning either at home or on the go. Serve cold.

Strawberries 'n' Dream Overnight Oats

SERVING SIZE: 1   **TOTAL TIME:** 5 minutes to prep, refrigerate overnight

Gluten-free, Vegetarian

½ cup rolled oats

¾ cup oat milk or
milk of choice

2 tablespoons chia seeds

¼ cup sliced fresh strawberries

¼ cup 2% plain Greek
or dairy-free yogurt

1 teaspoon vanilla extract

1. Combine your milk of choice with the oats in a mason jar.

2. Add the chia seeds, strawberries, Greek yogurt, and vanilla extract, and mix the ingredients together.

3. Seal with a lid and refrigerate overnight.

4. Enjoy the next morning either at home or on the go. Serve cold.

PB Chocolate Oat Milk Overnight Oats

SERVING SIZE: 1   **TOTAL TIME:** 5 minutes to prep, refrigerate overnight

Gluten-free, Dairy-free, Vegetarian

¾ cup oat milk or
milk of choice

½ cup rolled oats

2 tablespoons
chopped peanuts

1 tablespoon creamy
peanut butter

1 teaspoon maple syrup

½ teaspoon vanilla extract

¼ teaspoon unsweetened
cacao powder

1. Combine your milk of choice with the oats in a mason jar.

2. Add the peanuts, peanut butter, maple syrup, vanilla extract, and cacao powder, and mix the ingredients together.

3. Seal with a lid and refrigerate overnight.

4. Enjoy the next morning either at home or on the go. Serve cold.

Chunky Monkey Chia Seed Pudding

SERVING SIZE: 1   **TOTAL TIME:** 5 minutes to prep, refrigerate overnight

Gluten-free, Dairy-free, Vegetarian

1 banana, mashed

1 tablespoon almond butter

1 cup oat milk or milk of choice

3 tablespoons chia seeds

¼ teaspoon ground cinnamon

1 tablespoon flaxseeds or sunflower seeds, depending on the day of your cycle

1. Using a fork, combine the banana with the almond butter in a mason jar.

2. Add your choice of milk, chia seeds, cinnamon, and appropriate seeds, and mix the ingredients together.

3. Seal with a lid and refrigerate overnight.

4. Enjoy the next morning either at home or on the go. Serve cold.

No-Bake P.B.O. Energy Squares

SERVING SIZE: 16   **TOTAL TIME:** 20 minutes to prep, refrigerate 1 hour

Gluten-free, Dairy-free, Vegetarian

1 cup creamy peanut butter

½ cup maple syrup

2 cups rolled oats

½ cup dried raisins

½ cup chopped pistachios

½ teaspoon Himalayan salt

1. Line an 8-inch square baking pan with parchment paper, leaving extra paper hanging over two sides.

2. Lightly coat the parchment paper with cooking spray.

3. In a large bowl, mix the peanut butter and maple syrup. Stir in the oats, raisins, pistachios, and salt.

4. Spread the mixture firmly and distribute evenly in a baking pan.

5. Chill until firm, about 1 hour. Using extra parchment paper, lift the bars out of the baking pan.

6. Cut into 16 squares and serve.

Wild Blueberry Overnight Oats

SERVING SIZE: 2   **TOTAL TIME:** 10 minutes to prep, refrigerate overnight

Gluten-free, Dairy-free, Vegetarian

1 cup rolled oats

1¼ cups almond milk or milk of choice

4 tablespoons peanut butter

½ teaspoon ground cinnamon

2 teaspoons ground flaxseeds

2 teaspoons maple syrup

1 cup frozen blueberries

1. Combine the oats and milk of choice in a bowl until well mixed.

2. Add the peanut butter, cinnamon, flaxseeds, maple syrup, and blueberries, and mix well.

3. Divide the mixture between two mason jars or bowls with lids.

4. Cover with the lids and place in the refrigerator overnight.

5. Enjoy the next morning either at home or on the go. Serve cold.

Turmeric Avocado Toast with Sprouted Ezekiel Bread

SERVING SIZE: 2   **TOTAL TIME:** 10 minutes

Dairy-free, Vegetarian

4 slices sprouted Ezekiel bread or gluten-free bread

1 whole avocado, pitted and mashed

2 teaspoons Himalayan salt

⅛ teaspoon pepper

1 teaspoon garlic powder

1 whole medium tomato, sliced

1 teaspoon ground flaxseeds

2 tablespoons nutritional yeast

1 teaspoon ground turmeric

1 tablespoon Trader Joe's Everything But The Bagel Sesame Seasoning (or seasoning of choice)

1. Toast the bread in the oven at 350°F until crispy.

2. Mash the avocado with salt, pepper, and garlic powder.

3. Remove the bread and smear the avocado mash on top.

4. Top with the sliced tomato, flaxseeds, nutritional yeast, turmeric, and seasoning of choice.

Cinnamon Sweet Potato Yogurt Bowl

This bowl is a super-satisfying and healthy breakfast! You may be flocking toward lighter and brighter fare (thanks to the rising estrogen during the follicular phase), and the vibrant orange hues of a sweet potato definitely won't disappoint. These ingredients, though they may taste sweet, don't contain any refined sugar and are packed with fiber, vitamins A, C, and E, and iron coming from the sweet potato. Tip: Make the sweet potatoes ahead of time, then add them to your yogurt bowl in the morning.

SERVING SIZE: 2   **TOTAL TIME:** 35 minutes

Gluten-free, Vegetarian

1 sweet potato, diced

1 tablespoon avocado oil or olive oil

½ teaspoon ground cinnamon

1 cup plain Greek yogurt or dairy-free yogurt

1 large banana, sliced

4 tablespoons almond butter

1. Preheat the oven to 400°F.

2. Toss the sweet potato in the oil and cinnamon.

3. Spread onto a baking sheet lined with parchment paper in a single layer, and bake for 25 to 30 minutes. The sweet potatoes will be ready when a toothpick inserted in the middle comes out clean. Let cool.

4. To serve, put the yogurt in a bowl and top with the cooled sweet potatoes, sliced bananas, and almond butter.

Morning Honey Lemon Quinoa Parfait

This brekkie wakes up your taste buds in the morning, in the best way! Quinoa is a great plant-based protein option and the anti-inflammatory properties of honey can help with cramps. The chopped mint makes this parfait a super-refreshing, calming, and soothing way to start your morning, especially if PMS stress is coming in full swing.

SERVING SIZE: 2   **TOTAL TIME:** 25 minutes, including chill time

Gluten-free, Dairy-free, Vegetarian

1 cup fresh blueberries

1 cup sliced fresh strawberries

½ apple, chopped

1 cup cooked white, red, or tricolor quinoa

4 tablespoons chopped walnuts

2 tablespoons honey

juice of 1 lemon

1 teaspoon chopped fresh mint (optional)

1. Add all of the fruit, quinoa, and walnuts to a medium bowl, and gently mix together.

2. In a small bowl, stir the honey and lemon juice together to make a vinaigrette.

3. Pour the vinaigrette over the fruit salad and mix throughly.

4. Chill in the refrigerator for 10 minutes, then divide between 2 bowls and top with mint, if desired.

Vanilla-Spiced Date Caramel Sauce + Vanilla Yogurt

Now that you've satisfied your chocolate cravings, let this vanilla breakfast parfait excite your taste buds, stat! The vanilla notes deliver a delicious flavor profile so you won't be exhausted by all the chocolate (is that even possible!?). The probiotics in the yogurt will aid with any PMS-related bathroom issues and will keep your digestive system happy while the sunflower seeds, packed with vitamin E, will help relieve cramps.

SERVING SIZE: 2   **TOTAL TIME:** 15 minutes

Gluten-free, Vegetarian

8 to 10 pitted Medjool dates

4 tablespoons 88 Acres Vanilla Spiced Sunflower Seed Butter

1 teaspoon vanilla extract

1 teaspoon Himalayan salt

3 tablespoons unsweetened almond milk

1 cup vanilla Greek yogurt or vanilla dairy-free yogurt

2 tablespoons sunflower seeds

1. Place the dates, sunflower seed butter, vanilla extract, salt, and almond milk in a blender, and blend until smooth.

2. Divide the yogurt between 2 mason jars, drizzle the sauce on top, then sprinkle with sunflower seeds.

SNACKS

Spirulina Energy Balls

OVULATORY

Spirulina is a plant-based complete protein, meaning it contains 9 essential amino acids that keep our bodies healthy. It's also loaded with calcium, iron, magnesium, and vitamins A, E, and K. I like to snack on these energy balls around ovulation due to the helpful magnesium, antioxidants, and fiber properties, but they taste delicious (and are extremely nutritious), no matter the day of your cycle.

SERVING SIZE: 11 to 13   **TOTAL TIME:** 5 minutes plus 20 to 30 minutes chill time

Gluten-free, Dairy-free, Vegetarian

¾ cup rolled oats

½ cup pecans

2 teaspoons spirulina

1 cup soft pitted Medjool dates

2 tablespoons peanut butter

1. Add the oats, pecans, and spirulina to a high-speed blender or food processor and process until broken down.

2. Add the dates and peanut butter and process until a sticky dough forms.

3. Roll into balls about 2 inches thick and place on a parchment paper-lined baking sheet. Refrigerate for 20 to 30 minutes, until the texture has set.

4. Store in the refrigerator for 2 to 3 weeks or freezer for up to 6 months.

Apricot and Sunflower Energy Bites

SERVING SIZE: 10 to 12 balls   **TOTAL TIME:** 20 minutes, including chill time

Gluten-free, Dairy-free, Vegetarian

½ cup shredded
unsweetened coconut

1 teaspoon chia seeds

½ cup sunflower seeds

⅓ cup dried apricot

1½ tablespoons honey

small pinch of Himalayan salt

2 tablespoons cacao nibs

1. In a food processor, combine the coconut, chia seeds, and sunflower seeds, and pulse until ground.

2. Add the apricot and honey, and pulse until sticky.

3. Add a pinch of salt and cacao nibs to the food processor, and pulse 5 more times until fully combined.

4. Using the palms of your hands, roll into balls and refrigerate 10 minutes or until ready to serve.

Gluten-Free Peanut Butter Banana Bread

SERVING SIZE: 12   **TOTAL TIME:** 60 minutes

Gluten-free, Dairy-free, Vegetarian

⅛ teaspoon coconut oil

2 large ripe bananas, mashed

2 eggs

⅓ cup peanut butter

1 teaspoon vanilla extract

3 tablespoons applesauce

½ teaspoon baking soda

1 teaspoon baking powder

1 cup gluten-free flour

½ cup almond flour

½ cup coconut sugar

¼ teaspoon kosher salt

1. Preheat the oven to 350°F.

2. Lightly grease a bread pan with the coconut oil.

3. Add the bananas to a large mixing bowl, and mix in the eggs until frothy.

4. Mix in the peanut butter, vanilla, and applesauce.

5. Add the baking soda, baking powder, gluten-free flour, almond flour, sugar, and salt. Mix until just combined.

6. Pour the batter into the bread pan. Bake for 45 to 50 minutes (the top should be lightly browned and a toothpick should come out clean).

7. Remove from the oven and let cool for at least 10 minutes before slicing. Enjoy!

Crispy Chickpeas

SERVING SIZE: 2   **TOTAL TIME:** 35 minutes

Gluten-free, Dairy-free, Vegetarian

1 (15-ounce) can chickpeas, rinsed and drained

2 tablespoons olive oil

½ teaspoon smoked paprika

½ teaspoon garlic powder

⅛ teaspoon ground turmeric

½ teaspoon Himalayan salt

⅛ teaspoon cayenne pepper

1. Preheat the oven to 400°F, and line a rimmed baking sheet with parchment paper.

2. Pour the chickpeas onto a clean kitchen towel or paper towel, and thoroughly pat dry.

3. Spread the chickpeas on the baking sheet, and toss with the oil, paprika, garlic powder, turmeric, salt, and cayenne pepper. Spread evenly in a single layer.

4. Bake for 20 minutes, shake, and then return to the oven for another 10 minutes, or until crispy.

5. Allow the chickpeas to cool completely prior to serving. The chickpeas can be used as a snack or on top of salads.

Honey Turmeric Nuts

Elevate your snacks by simply roasting anti-inflammatory whole nuts with honey, pepper, and turmeric. Choose your favorite nuts but don't forget to include peanuts. Peanuts are a powerful source of healthy unsaturated fat and B vitamins, which help promote progesterone production and estrogen balance in the body. Turmeric's antioxidant and inflammation-fighting power will also help to squash cramps in both the PMS and menstrual phase, making you feel energized and pain-free. Bonus: Pairing the turmeric with pepper will allow the anti-inflammatory compounds in turmeric to soar by up to 2,000%. Talk about a healthy dynamic duo!

SERVING SIZE: 8   **TOTAL TIME:** 15 minutes

Gluten-free, Dairy-free, Vegetarian

3½ cups whole, raw nuts (choose your favorites: peanuts, cashews, almonds, hazelnuts, macadamia nuts, walnuts, pecans, pistachios)

2 tablespoons honey

2 tablespoons coconut oil or olive oil

1 teaspoon ground turmeric

½ teaspoon ground cinnamon

½ teaspoon sea salt

⅛ teaspoon black pepper

⅛ teaspoon cayenne pepper (optional)

1. Preheat the oven to 350°F. Line a rimmed baking sheet with parchment paper.

2. In a large bowl, combine the nuts, honey, and oil. Sprinkle the turmeric, cinnamon, salt, pepper, and cayenne pepper, if using, over the mixture, and toss to coat.

3. Spread the nuts on the baking sheet and roast in the center of the oven for 8 to 12 minutes, stirring every 4 minutes until the nuts are aromatic and slightly darker.

4. Allow to cool completely before serving. Store in a mason jar or airtight container for up to 2 weeks.

Rosemary Roasted Walnuts

SERVING SIZE: 4 (¼-cup) servings   **TOTAL TIME:** 15 minutes

Gluten-free, Dairy-free, Vegetarian

1 cup walnuts, kept whole

1 tablespoon coconut oil

½ tablespoon finely chopped fresh rosemary

¼ teaspoon sea salt

1. Preheat the oven to 350°F and line a baking sheet with parchment paper.

2. Toss the walnuts, coconut oil, rosemary, and salt in a medium bowl until the walnuts are covered in oil. Evenly distribute on the prepared baking sheet.

3. Bake about 10 to 15 minutes until the walnuts are fragrant and golden brown, tossing every 5 minutes so they don't burn.

4. Allow to cool completely before serving. Store in a mason jar or airtight container for up to 2 weeks.

Chocolate Zucchini Smoothie

A delicious low-sugar smoothie indeed! Zucchini is very hydrating, which will help decrease any PMS-related bloat. Tip: Steam your zucchini ahead of time so it's easier to digest. Then freeze the zucchini to make this smoothie thick, creamy, and nutritious.

SERVING SIZE: 1   **TOTAL TIME:** 5 minutes

Gluten-free, Dairy-free, Vegetarian

1 cup soy milk or milk of choice

2 cups fresh or frozen baby kale or spinach

½ frozen banana

½ cup frozen zucchini

2 tablespoons nut butter of choice

½ teaspoon spirulina

½ teaspoon cacao powder

1. Combine all the ingredients in a blender and blend at high speed until completely smooth.

2. Enjoy immediately.

Tropical Green Smoothie

SERVING SIZE: 1   **TOTAL TIME:** 5 minutes

Gluten-free, Dairy-free, Vegetarian

2 cups frozen spinach	½ cup frozen pineapple
1 tablespoon ground flaxseeds	1 cup soy milk or milk of choice
1 frozen banana	1 teaspoon spirulina
½ cup papaya	½ cup ice

1. Combine all the ingredients in a blender and blend for 30 to 60 seconds until you reach the desired consistency.

2. Enjoy immediately.

Pretty Pretty Chocolate Pumpkin Morning Muffins

SERVING SIZE: 24 mini muffins or 12 regular muffins **TOTAL TIME:** 40 minutes

Gluten-free, Vegetarian

1 cup oat flour*

½ teaspoon baking powder

½ cup 88 Acres Pumpkin Seed Butter

1 egg

½ cup unsweetened applesauce

½ cup pumpkin puree

1 teaspoon vanilla extract

½ cup dark chocolate chips, or dairy-free dark chocolate chips

pumpkin seeds, for topping (optional)

1. Preheat the oven to 350°F. Line a muffin tin with liners or grease with oil, and set aside.

2. In a large bowl, combine the oat flour and baking powder, and set aside. In a medium bowl, mix pumpkin seed butter, egg, applesauce, pumpkin puree, and vanilla extract until well combined.

3. Add the wet ingredients to the dry ingredients and stir gently until fully incorporated. Sprinkle in the dark chocolate chips, and stir to combine.

4. Portion out into muffin tins and fill each mold about three-quarters full. Top with the pumpkin seeds, if desired.

5. Bake for 15 to 20 minutes, or until the tops are lightly golden and firm to the touch. Let cool completely before serving.

* To make your own oat flour, pulse rolled oats in a food processor until pulverized into a flour.

TIPS: Try adding butternut squash puree, shredded zucchini, grated carrots, or pureed spinach for a micronutrient boost.

Choco-Nutty Monkey Smoothie

LUTEAL/PMS

SERVING SIZE: 2   **TOTAL TIME:** 10 minutes

Gluten-free, Dairy-free, Vegetarian

2 cups almond milk
or milk of choice

2 cups fresh or frozen spinach

½ cup frozen cauliflower

2 tablespoons almond butter

1 frozen banana

1 tablespoon cacao powder

1 tablespoon cacao nibs

handful of ice (for
an icier texture)

1 tablespoon cacao
nibs, for garnish

1. Add all the ingredients to the blender, and blend on high until smooth.

2. Sprinkle with cacao nibs and serve.

Sweet Pea Hummus

MENSTRUAL, FOLLICULAR, OVULATORY

Making your own hummus has never been so easy and nutritious! Although it may seem intimidating at first, it's great to have the option of adding your own favorite and healing ingredients like garlic, antioxidants from lime, and a burst of flavor from red pepper flakes. You won't disappoint your taste buds! Plus, let tahini, a ground sesame paste, be your secret weapon as it contains magnesium, known to help stabilize mood and decrease anxiety as hormones rise and fall throughout the cycle.

SERVING SIZE: 8   **TOTAL TIME:** 10 minutes

Gluten-free, Dairy-free, Vegetarian

4 cloves garlic, minced

2 cups sweet peas, frozen + thawed for 5 minutes

1 (28-ounce) can chickpeas, rinsed and drained

½ lime, squeezed

3 tablespoons olive oil

1 tablespoon tahini

red pepper flakes, to garnish

sprouts, microgreens, or pesto, to garnish (optional)

sea salt and pepper

1. In a food processor or high-speed blender process the minced garlic and sweet peas until they form a paste-like consistency.

2. Add the chickpeas, lime juice, olive oil, and tahini.

3. Blend until smooth, scraping down the edges as needed.

4. Season with salt and pepper to taste. Garnish with the red pepper flakes and other desired toppings. Serve with crudités.

Gluten-Free Pumpkin Bread

SERVING SIZE: 12   **TOTAL TIME:** 60 minutes

Gluten-free, Dairy-free, Vegetarian

⅛ teaspoon coconut oil

1½ cups almond flour

¼ cup gluten-free flour

¾ teaspoon baking soda

1 teaspoon ground cinnamon

¼ teaspoon nutmeg

½ teaspoon pumpkin pie spice

¼ teaspoon ground ginger

½ teaspoon kosher salt

2 tablespoons coconut sugar

¾ cup pumpkin puree

¼ cup maple syrup

2 eggs

1. Preheat the oven to 350°F.

2. Lightly grease a bread pan with the coconut oil.

3. Combine all the dry ingredients (almond flour through coconut sugar).

4. In a separate bowl, combine the wet ingredients (pumpkin puree, maple syrup, and eggs).

5. Add the wet ingredients to the dry ingredients and mix until combined.

6. Pour the batter into the bread pan.

7. Bake for approximately 40 minutes until the top is lightly browned and a toothpick will come out clean.

8. Let the bread stand in the pan for at least 10 minutes.

9. Transfer to a cooling rack and cool completely before serving.

Maple Seed Butter-Glazed Carrots

OVULATORY, LUTEAL/PMS

This side dish is overflowing with nutritious beta-carotene, a superstar orange pigment that's been touted for its antioxidant and immune-boosting properties. As your cycle progresses past the menstrual phase, you can become more susceptible to infection as the body works tirelessly to rebuild a healthy endometrial lining. Carrots help to keep your immune system strong so you can keep chugging along, without any colds or sicknesses in sight! If you want to elevate your carrot game, look for heirloom carrots (purple, white, yellow) for a fancy pop of color. The carrots also work in both the ovulatory and luteal phase to provide your ovaries with antioxidant protection while it releases a follicle and to keep your uterus and fallopian tubes healthy in case conception is in cards!

SERVING SIZE: 2   **TOTAL TIME:** 1 hour

Gluten-free, Dairy-free, Vegetarian

ROASTED CARROTS

8 small carrots, peeled

2 tablespoons olive oil

⅛ teaspoon salt

⅛ teaspoon pepper

2 tablespoons chopped flat-leaf parsley or chives (optional)

MAPLE GLAZE

¼ cup 88 Acres Maple Sunflower Seed Butter

1 tablespoon maple syrup

¼ teaspoon salt

⅛ teaspoon pepper

pinch of nutmeg

warm water, to thin

1. Preheat the oven to 400°F and coat a baking sheet with cooking spray.

2. In a medium bowl, toss together the peeled carrots, olive oil, salt, and pepper until evenly coated. Arrange in a single layer on the prepared baking sheet.

3. Roast for 25 to 30 minutes, until the carrots are tender. Start checking for doneness after 15 to 20 minutes if your carrots are on the smaller side.

4. While the carrots are roasting, prepare the Maple Glaze. In a medium bowl, add all the ingredients except for the water, and whisk to combine. Slowly stream in the warm water while whisking until the maple glaze reaches a drizzling consistency. Set aside.

5. To serve, arrange the carrots on a serving dish with stems on one side. Drizzle the maple glaze lightly over the carrots and garnish with fresh herbs like parsley or chives, if desired.

6. Serve the remaining glaze on the side.

7. Pair with soups, grains, burgers, fish, or chicken.

Parm Cheese and Broccoli Pasta

SERVING SIZE: 2   **TOTAL TIME:** 30 minutes

Vegetarian

3 cups broccoli, chopped into florets

2 tablespoons olive oil

⅛ cup Italian-style or gluten-free breadcrumbs

¼ cup freshly shredded Parmesan cheese or nutritional yeast if dairy-free, plus more to serve

1 teaspoon garlic powder

¼ teaspoon salt

pinch of pepper

½ box bean-based or whole grain pasta

1. Preheat the oven to 425°F.

2. Add the water to a medium saucepan over medium heat.

3. Line a baking sheet with tinfoil and nonstick cooking spray.

4. In a medium bowl, combine the broccoli, olive oil, breadcrumbs, Parmesan cheese, garlic powder, salt, and pepper, and mix to coat.

5. Spread the coated broccoli onto the baking sheet.

6. Bake for 12 minutes then flip the broccoli and bake for another 10 minutes, until crispy.

7. In the meantime, once water is boiling, add the pasta to a saucepan and cook according to the box directions.

8. Combine the cooked pasta and cooked crispy broccoli in bowl and sprinkle Parmesan cheese on top.

Creamy Roasted Garlic and Cauliflower Soup

As hormones tend to rise and fall mid-cycle, it's essential to take care of a vital organ that helps with the metabolism, breakdown, and excretion of hormones–the liver! To help support the hard-working liver, choose allium-rich vegetables, such as onion and garlic. Plus, sulfur-rich foods, like cauliflower, are filled with glutathione, an antioxidant that assists with liver detoxification. This soup blends together these helpful ingredients so your liver works like a well-oiled machine.

SERVING SIZE: 4   **TOTAL TIME:** 1 hour 10 minutes

Gluten-free, Dairy-free, Vegetarian

1 small head garlic

2 medium heads cauliflower, chopped into florets

5 tablespoons olive oil, divided

1 sprig fresh rosemary, finely chopped

1 small onion, diced

1 pinch red pepper flakes

1 (15-ounce) can white beans, drained and rinsed

1 quart vegetable broth

1 cup unsweetened, unflavored almond milk

kosher salt

black pepper

1. Preheat the oven to 400°F.

2. Cut off the top of the head of garlic so the cloves are exposed and place in the center of a baking sheet.

3. Spread the cauliflower florets around the garlic.

4. Drizzle the garlic head and cauliflower with 4 tablespoons of olive oil and then sprinkle with the salt, pepper, and chopped rosemary.

5. Wrap the garlic head in foil and roast everything in the oven for 30 minutes.

6. When the roasting is complete, add the remaining tablespoon of olive oil to a large soup pot over medium heat.

7. Wait 1 minute, then add the diced onion and red pepper flakes to the soup pot. Cook until the onions become translucent and fragrant, about 3 to 4 minutes.

8. Remove the whole roasted garlic cloves from the garlic head (be careful not to burn yourself!), and add the cloves to the pot with the rosemary-roasted cauliflower, white beans, vegetable broth, and milk, and bring to a boil. Add a dash of salt and pepper to taste.

9. Reduce to a simmer and cook for 30 minutes. Use a blender to puree the soup until creamy. Add more salt and pepper to taste. If too thick, add more milk to adjust consistency.

10. Enjoy while hot!

Coconut-Infused Butternut Squash Soup

SERVING SIZE: 2   **TOTAL TIME:** 40 minutes

Gluten-free, Dairy-free, Vegetarian

½ tablespoon olive oil

½ medium diced yellow onion

2 cloves garlic, minced

1 teaspoon grated fresh ginger

½ teaspoon kosher salt

⅛ teaspoon pepper

½ teaspoon dried thyme

½ medium butternut squash, peeled and cubed

2 cups vegetable stock

½ cup unflavored coconut milk

2 fresh thyme sprigs, to garnish

2 tablespoons coconut yogurt, to garnish

1. Place a large saucepan on medium heat.

2. Add the olive oil, onion, garlic, ginger, salt, pepper, and thyme, and cook until the onion becomes translucent, about 4 to 5 minutes. Be careful not to burn.

3. Add the cubed butternut squash and stock to the mixture. The broth should sit under the squash, so add more or less broth based on the level.

4. Cover the pot and bring to a boil at medium high.

5. Once the soup boils, turn down to medium and let simmer for about 20 minutes or until you can pierce the squash with a fork.

6. Remove the soup from the heat and add the coconut milk.

7. Either blend until smooth with an immersion blender OR blend in a Vitamix or high-speed blender for about 30 seconds.

8. Serve immediately and top with thyme and coconut yogurt with your favorite crackers on the side.

Peaches and Cream Toast

Elevate your lunch game with this tasty toast creation! The best part about this toast is that the peaches are so soft and juicy to begin with, you don't even have to bake them to create this masterpiece—literally just slice and layer! It's best to eat this in the luteal phase to gain the vitamin D and magnesium benefits in the Greek yogurt and to enjoy the natural sugars from the peach and honey.

SERVING SIZE: 1   **TOTAL TIME:** 5 minutes

Gluten-free, Vegetarian

2 slices gluten-free or sprouted bread

½ cup 2% plain Greek or dairy-free yogurt

½ peach, sliced

88 Acres Seed'nola blend or your favorite gluten-free granola

1 tablespoon honey

1. Toast the bread.

2. Top with yogurt, peach slices, and granola, and drizzle with some raw honey.

Sweet Potato Avocado Rice Bowl

This is a dream lunch for me as it contains all the ingredients my taste buds and my hormones want. This bowl compiles healthy components coming from heart-protecting unsaturated fat, belly-filling fiber, and energizing iron. Because it uses cilantro, it helps to scale down the sodium so you'll feel less bloated afterward. Plus, it is packed with protein coming from the Banza chickpea rice, a rich, plant-based source of protein that contains way less carbs, and much more fiber and protein than regular white rice. This bowl will keep you satisfied for long periods of time, so you can rechannel your energy toward more enticing behaviors (such as intercourse) during ovulation.

SERVING SIZE: 4   **TOTAL TIME:** 30 minutes

Gluten-free, Vegetarian

2 large sweet potatoes, peeled and cut into 1-inch cubes

4 tablespoons olive oil, divided, plus more for serving

½ teaspoon Himalayan salt

pepper

¼ cup pumpkin seeds

4 ounces feta or dairy-free cheese, drained

1 bag Banza chickpea rice

½ cup coarsely chopped fresh cilantro leaves

zest of 2 medium limes

juice of 2 medium limes, plus more wedges to serve

1 medium avocado, pitted and quartered

1. Arrange 2 racks to divide the oven into thirds, and preheat to 425°F. Place the sweet potatoes on a baking sheet covered with tinfoil or parchment paper.

2. Drizzle with 2 tablespoons of oil, then season with the salt and pepper to taste. Toss to combine, then arrange into an even layer. Roast on the lower rack until the sweet potatoes begin to brown, about 20 minutes.

3. Flip the sweet potatoes and push them to one side. Add the pumpkin seeds to the now-empty portion of the baking sheet and crumble the feta into large pieces over the sweet potatoes. Roast until the pumpkin seeds are toasted, the sweet potatoes are golden-brown, and the feta is warmed through, 5 to 7 minutes.

4. Meanwhile, in a medium saucepan, cook the Banza rice according to package instructions, strain, and rinse. Add it back to the saucepan and add cilantro, lime zest, lime juice, remaining 2 tablespoon oil, salt, and several grinds of pepper. Toss until evenly coated; set aside.

5. For each serving: transfer ¼ of the rice and ¼ of the sweet potato and feta mixture. Sprinkle with ¼ of the pepitas and top with a piece of the avocado (peel the avocado if eating immediately). Drizzle with more olive oil and season with salt and pepper as needed. Serve with a lime wedge.

Bok Choy and Tofu

SERVING SIZE: 2   **TOTAL TIME:** 50 minutes

Gluten-free, Dairy-free, Vegetarian

6 ounces extra-firm tofu, drained

1 tablespoon sesame oil

1 tablespoon cornstarch

1 large clove garlic, minced

½ tablespoon ginger, minced

½ tablespoon rice vinegar

2 tablespoons coconut sugar

1½ teaspoons + 1½ tablespoons tamari, divided

¼ cup almond milk

½ tablespoon water

1 tablespoon garlic chili sauce

½ teaspoon toasted sesame oil

½ tablespoon maple syrup

1 tablespoon avocado oil

4 whole bok choy heads, split horizontally

2 tablespoons sesame seeds, to serve

1. Preheat the oven to 375°F.

2. Wrap the tofu in an absorbent towel and put something heavy on top to remove the moisture. Let sit for 20 to 25 minutes.

3. Make the sauce by combining the sesame oil, cornstarch, garlic, ginger, rice vinegar, coconut sugar, 1½ teaspoons tamari, almond milk, and water in a bowl, and whisk until combined with no clumps. Set aside.

4. Unwrap and cut the tofu into even, ¾-inch cubes.

5. Add the tofu to a bowl and mix with the remaining tamari, chili garlic sauce, sesame oil, and maple syrup, and toss to combine. Let it sit for a few minutes, mixing occasionally.

6. Place a large skillet over medium heat. Add avocado oil to the skillet and warm through for 2 to 3 minutes. Add the tofu to the pan, and flip every minute until slightly cooked, about 5 minutes.

Remove pan from stove top and place in the oven for 15 minutes or until crispy.

7. While the tofu is cooking, add water to medium saucepan and heat over medium-high heat. Once the water is boiling, reduce heat to medium-low heat and, using steamer basket, steam the bok choy for about 6 minutes until fork tender. Remove and set aside.

8. Remove the tofu and place the skillet back on the burner over medium heat. Add the bok choy, tofu, and sauce back into the pan and mix together until warm.

9. Remove and serve with sesame seeds. Completely the meal with your choice of 1 cup brown rice, quinoa, or cauliflower rice.

Eggocado Open-Faced Sandy

SERVING SIZE: 2   **TOTAL TIME:** 10 minutes

Gluten-free, Vegetarian

3 hard-boiled eggs, peeled, quartered, and chopped in pieces

1 avocado, halved and pitted

2 tablespoons plus 1 tablespoon coarsely chopped fresh basil leaves, divided

2 tablespoons thinly sliced scallions

½ teaspoon ground turmeric

1 tablespoon 2 or 4% plain Greek yogurt or dairy-free yogurt

½ teaspoon lemon juice

pinch of kosher salt

pinch of pepper

2 slices sprouted bread or gluten-free bread, toasted

2 tablespoons thinly sliced radishes (roughly 4 radishes)

1. Place the eggs in a medium bowl.

2. Scoop out the avocado flesh and add it to the bowl. Mash the eggs and avocado lightly with a fork, maintaining a chunky texture.

3. Add the basil, scallions, turmeric, yogurt, lemon juice, a pinch of salt, and a pinch of pepper. Gently mix until all of the ingredients are incorporated. Taste and adjust the seasonings as needed.

4. Divide the egg salad among the toasted bread slices, spreading into an even layer.

5. Garnish with the remaining basil and thinly sliced radishes, and serve.

Moroccan Quinoa Salad

SERVING SIZE: 3   **TOTAL TIME:** 55 minutes

Gluten-free, Dairy-free, Vegetarian

SALAD

1 (15-ounce) can chickpeas, drained and rinsed

4 tablespoons olive oil, divided

½ tablespoon Himalayan salt

¼ tablespoon pepper

1 cup dry quinoa

2 cups water

4 large carrots, peeled and diced

2 cloves garlic, minced

1 jar roasted bell peppers (typically contains 2 to 3 large bell peppers), drained and diced

⅓ cup raisins

DRESSING

½ cup white balsamic vinegar

4 tablespoons olive oil, divided

1 tablespoon honey (optional)

¼ cup chopped flat-leaf parsley

2 teaspoons ground turmeric

1 teaspoon ground cumin

Himalayan salt, to taste

pepper, to taste

1. Preheat the oven to 450°F.

2. Spread the chickpeas evenly onto a rimmed baking sheet and sprinkle with 3 tablespoons of olive oil, salt, and black pepper. Roast in the oven until crisp, about 30 minutes, rotating every 10 minutes to prevent burning.

3. Meanwhile, add the quinoa and water to a medium saucepan. Bring to a boil over high heat then reduce heat to low, cover, and simmer for about 15 minutes until the water is absorbed.

4. Add the carrots, garlic, and 1 tablespoon of olive oil to a large sauté pan over medium heat and cook until the carrots are tender, roughly 5 minutes.

5. Add the roasted bell peppers and raisins to the sauté pan and cook until warm, about 3 minutes.

6. Add the cooked quinoa to the sauté pan, and toss the quinoa salad with the dressing ingredients.

7. Sprinkle the roasted chickpeas on top of the quinoa salad. Enjoy warm or cool.

Smashed Potatoes with Garlic Pumpkin Seed Pesto

You naturally have plenty of energy during ovulation, and potatoes continue to help fuel this natural boost! Because potatoes are rich in potassium, which help fluids become evenly dispersed throughout the body, you will be less likely to feel bloated and more likely to feel your absolute best during this phase! Plus, the pesto contains nutritional yeast, which is loaded with vitamin B12, known to help keep energy levels up, up, up!

SERVING SIZE: 2 **TOTAL TIME:** 1 hour

Gluten-free, Dairy-free, Vegetarian

POTATOES

1½ pounds baby gold or yellow potatoes

1½ tablespoons olive oil

½ teaspoon salt

⅛ teaspoon pepper

GARLIC PUMPKIN SEED PESTO

2 cups fresh basil, loosely packed

1 tablespoon 88 Acres Pumpkin Seed Butter

2 cloves garlic, peeled

2 tablespoons lemon juice

1½ tablespoons nutritional yeast

1 tablespoon olive oil

¼ teaspoon salt

⅛ teaspoon pepper

1. Preheat the oven to 450°F and prepare a baking sheet with parchment paper.

2. Place the potatoes in a large pot and fill with water until potatoes are just submerged. Bring to a boil over high heat, then reduce to medium and simmer for 15 to 20 minutes, or until potatoes are fork-tender.

3. Drain the potatoes and remove from the heat. Arrange potatoes on the prepared baking sheet, leaving space between each potato. Using a heavy-bottomed saucepan, gently press each potato until flattened to roughly ½ inch in height. Drizzle each smashed potato with olive oil and season generously with salt and pepper. Roast for 15 to 20 minutes, until edges are golden brown.

4. While potatoes are roasting, add the pesto ingredients to a food processor, and pulse until combined and smooth.

5. Transfer the potatoes to a serving dish and top with a drizzle of Garlic Pumpkin Seed Pesto. Serve with your favorite protein and with leftover pesto on the side.

Tahini, Kale, and Farro Stuffed Sweet Potatoes

SERVING SIZE: 3   **TOTAL TIME:** 60 minutes

Dairy-free, Vegetarian

SWEET POTATOES

3 medium sweet potatoes

1 cup farro, or quinoa
if gluten-free

2 cups vegetable broth

1 tablespoon olive oil

4 cups chopped kale

TAHINI SAUCE

3 cloves garlic, crushed

1 cup tahini

½ cup flat-leaf parsley,
stems removed

⅓ cup lemon juice

¼ cup olive oil

1 cup warm water

⅛ teaspoon Himalayan
salt, plus more to taste

1. Preheat the oven to 425°F.

2. Poke a few holes in the sweet potatoes and place them on a baking sheet lined with parchment paper. Bake for 45 to 55 minutes, until soft to touch. Set aside to cool.

3. While sweet potatoes are cooking, in a small pot, add the farro and vegetable broth. Bring to a boil and then cover and reduce heat to a simmer. Simmer for up to 40 minutes, until grains are tender and have absorbed all of the liquid.

4. In a food processor or high-speed blender, add all the tahini sauce ingredients and process until creamy. Taste and add salt, if needed.

5. Drizzle the olive oil In a medium saucepan over medium heat. When hot, add the kale and sauté until crispy.

6. Mix the cooked farro, crispy kale, and a few spoonfuls of tahini together until lightly coated.

7. Cut the sweet potatoes open in the center lengthwise and spoon the farro mixture into the middle of each sweet potato. Add an extra drizzle of tahini sauce on top.

Edamame Pesto and Goat Cheese Toast

SERVING SIZE: 1   **TOTAL TIME:** 10 minutes

Vegetarian

1 cup shelled edamame (defrost if frozen), plus more for garnish

2 teaspoons minced garlic

2 cups shredded fresh basil leaves

¼ cup olive oil

juice from ½ lemon

½ teaspoon Himalayan salt

pinch of pepper

1 slice Ezekiel sprouted bread or gluten-free bread, toasted

¼ cup sliced cucumber, to top

¼ cup halved cherry tomatoes, to top

2 tablespoons goat cheese or dairy-free cheese, to top

1. Add the edamame, garlic, basil, olive oil, lemon juice, salt, and pepper to a food processor, and process until fairly smooth (it won't get perfectly smooth).

2. Spread the edamame pesto over the toast.

3. Top with sliced cucumber, halved cherry tomatoes, goat cheese, a few shelled edamame pieces, and a sprinkle of salt and pepper.

Pineapple Cauliflower Fried Rice

A new spin on fried rice, subbing in cauliflower for white rice not only reduces the refined carbohydrates but also keeps blood sugar spikes to a minimum thanks to fiber. Expect to feel energized, nourished, and refreshed after this dish and I promise, you won't even miss the rice! Cauliflower provides vitamin C, which helps the body absorb more iron, a nutrient that is often quite low during menstruation. Therefore, this dish is good during PMS to help pump up the iron before menstruation hits. Also, vitamin C is integral to healthy ovulation and vitamin C tends to dip low before and during ovulation. That's why this recipe is also great to have during ovulation to ensure a successful ovulation cycle.

SERVING SIZE: 2   **TOTAL TIME:** 20 minutes

Gluten-free, Dairy-free, Vegetarian

3 (omega-3-enriched) eggs

¼ teaspoon Himalayan salt

2 tablespoons olive oil, divided

2 teaspoons toasted sesame oil, divided

2 cups diced fresh pineapple

1 large diced bell pepper

2 medium carrots, diced

½ cup shelled edamame (thawed if frozen)

3 thinly sliced scallions

2 cloves garlic, minced

1 medium head cauliflower, shredded or pulsed in a food processor until it resembles small grains of rice, or riced cauliflower (fresh or frozen)

2 tablespoons coconut aminos

2 teaspoons sriracha sauce

1 tablespoon ground flaxseeds

1 sunny-side up egg, to top, optional

1. In a small bowl, whisk the eggs with the salt.

2. In a large nonstick skillet, heat 1 tablespoon of olive oil. Once the oil is hot and shiny, about 2 minutes, add the eggs and cook, stirring occasionally, until barely set. Transfer to a large, clean bowl and toss with 1 teaspoon of sesame oil.

3. Carefully wipe the skillet clean, then heat the remaining tablespoon of olive oil over medium-high. Add the pineapple, bell pepper, and carrots. Cook, stirring constantly, until the juices have evaporated and the pineapple is lightly caramelized, 8 to 10 minutes.

4. Stir in the edamame, scallions, and garlic, and cook until fragrant, 30 seconds to 1 minute.

5. Add the cauliflower to the skillet. Cook until the cauliflower is hot but not mushy, 1 to 2 minutes. Stir in the cooked eggs, coconut aminos, sriracha sauce, and remaining 1 teaspoon sesame oil.

6. Top with scallions, flaxseeds, and a sunny-side-up egg, if desired. Serve warm.

DINNER

Loaded Spaghetti Squash Boats

Not only will this dinner impress the heck out of all your Instagram followers when you put it on your story, but it will help to keep your body calm and happy during your cycle, no matter the phase. Spaghetti squash will nourish and heal your body as it helps to replenish iron, antioxidants, and vitamins A, C, and E, all needed to support a healthy menstrual cycle which is why it's great any day! In fact, spaghetti squash is loaded with vitamin A, which assists in healthy ovulation. Bonus: The pine nuts are nutritional powerhouses, providing a hefty amount of relaxing magnesium, shown to reduce cramps by soothing muscle contractions in the uterus. Double bonus: Magnesium can also aid in sleep, help to lower stress, and aid in the production of progesterone.

SERVING SIZE: 2   **TOTAL TIME:** 1 hour

Gluten-free, Vegetarian

1 tablespoon olive oil

1 medium-sized spaghetti squash, cut lengthwise and seeds scraped

½ teaspoon salt

¼ teaspoon pepper

4 cups of your favorite marinara sauce

½ cup shredded part-skim or whole milk mozzarella cheese or dairy-free cheese

4 tablespoons pine nuts

1. Preheat the oven to 400°F.

2. Rub the olive oil inside each squash half, and season with salt and pepper.

3. Place the squash face-down in a large baking dish and bake for 50 minutes, until the squash is fork-tender.

4. Remove the baking dish from the oven and turn to broil. Using a fork, scrape the spaghetti squash so its strands become separated. Make a shallow pocket in the middle of each boat and pour marinara sauce into each squash half.

5. Top each squash "boat" with ¼ cup cheese.

6. Once the broiler is ready, place the baking dish with assembled squash boats into oven for 3 to 4 minutes or until cheese turns brown.

7. Sprinkle the pine nuts on top of each squash boat and enjoy warm!

Butternut Squash and Kale Frittata

SERVING SIZE: 6   **TOTAL TIME:** 45 minutes

Gluten-free, Vegetarian

2 cups butternut squash, cubed

4 tablespoons olive oil, divided

Himalayan salt, to taste

pinch of pepper, to taste

8 to 10 (omega-3–enriched) eggs

½ red onion, diced

1 whole yellow bell pepper, diced

3 handfuls of raw chopped kale

½ cup goat cheese or dairy-free cheese

1. Preheat the oven to 400°F.

2. Toss the butternut squash in 2 tablespoons olive oil, salt, and pepper, and bake for about 30 minutes until fork tender.

3. Crack the eggs into a medium bowl and whisk with a dash of salt and pepper. Set aside.

4. Add 2 tablespoons olive oil to a medium oven-safe skillet over medium heat.

5. Add the onion and pepper, and sauté 5 minutes until tender.

6. Add the kale, and sauté until tender.

7. Add the roasted butternut squash to the skillet, a few dashes of salt and pepper, and mix together.

8. Pour the eggs into the skillet and turn the heat to medium-low.

9. Cook until the top starts to set, but there is still some liquid on the top, 4 to 5 minutes.

10. Sprinkle the crumbled goat cheese on top.

11. Turn the broiler on high and place the skillet in the oven for 3 to 4 minutes until the top is completely set and slightly browned.

Rotisserie Chicken Detox Salad

SERVING SIZE: 2   **TOTAL TIME:** 25 minutes

Gluten-free

SALAD

2 cups almonds

2 cups chopped kale

1 tablespoon olive oil

2 cups shredded Brussels sprouts

1 cup shredded store-bought rotisserie chicken, sub for 1 cup white beans if vegetarian

½ cup feta or dairy-free cheese, crumbled

¼ cup sunflower seeds

VINAIGRETTE

2 tablespoons lemon juice

½ tablespoon apple cider vinegar

⅛ cup olive oil

½ tablespoon Dijon mustard

½ teaspoon minced garlic

1 teaspoon salt

1 teaspoon nutritional yeast

1. Preheat the oven to 350°F. Spread the almonds on a baking sheet (do not overlap).

2. Bake for 5 minutes and stir. Continue to bake until fragrant, another 2 to 3 minutes. Do not burn!

3. Put chopped kale in a large bowl and mix with olive oil. Massage with hands until soft.

4. Add Brussels sprouts to large bowl with kale, and let sit.

5. Mix all the vinaigrette ingredients together in a medium bowl.

6. Drizzle dressing over Brussel sprouts and kale. Add the shredded chicken, feta, sunflower seeds, and toasted almonds. Mix together.

7. Chill in the refrigerator until ready to serve.

Pumpkin Pesto Pasta

SERVING SIZE: 2   **TOTAL TIME:** 20 minutes

Gluten-free, Vegetarian

½ box rotini Banza pasta

½ packed cup frozen spinach, thawed for 10 minutes

¼ packed cup fresh basil

3 tablespoons 88 Acres Pumpkin Seed Butter with no added sugar

3 tablespoons Parmesan cheese or nutritional yeast if dairy-free, plus more for garnish

3 tablespoons lemon juice

pinch of salt

pinch of pepper

¼ cup olive oil, divided

1. Cook the rotini according to package instructions. Once cooked, rinse with cold water and drain.

2. While the pasta cooks, about 10 minutes, place the thawed spinach, basil, pumpkin seed butter, cheese or yeast, lemon juice, salt, pepper, and half of the olive oil in a food processor.

3. Blend everything together while drizzling the remaining olive oil into the food processor until the pesto reaches a smooth consistency.

4. Combine the pesto and Banza pasta in a bowl, sprinkling additional Parmesan cheese on top.

Sweet Potato Tacos

SERVING SIZE: 3   **TOTAL TIME:** 25 minutes

Gluten-free, Dairy-free, Vegetarian

2 tablespoons olive oil

2 large sweet potatoes, peeled and chopped into small, ½-inch pieces

pinch of Himalayan salt and pepper

½ teaspoon ground cumin

1 teaspoon minced garlic

¾ cup canned black beans, drained and rinsed

3 gluten-free tortillas (coconut, corn, cassava, almond, or cashew)

store-bought pico de gallo

1 avocado, sliced

1 jalapeño, sliced (optional)

1. Drizzle the olive oil in a nonstick skillet over medium heat. Warm for 2 minutes.

2. Add the sweet potatoes, salt, pepper, and cumin. Sauté for about 10 to 15 minutes until the sweet potato is tender and begins to brown.

3. Add the garlic, black beans, and another dash of salt and pepper, and sauté for another minute or so until the garlic is fragrant and the black beans are warm.

4. Broil the tortillas in the oven on low until warm.

5. Top each tortilla with the sweet potato mixture, pico de gallo, a few slices of avocado, and jalapeño.

Quinoa-Stuffed Acorn Squash

As your body gears up for PMS and menstruation, you want all the iron, vitamins A, C, and E, and antioxidants your body can handle to keep inflammation and pain at bay. This dinner delivers on all accounts, providing nutritional benefits coming from the quinoa, acorn squash, and kale so it's great for the luteal phase and during PMS.

SERVING SIZE: 4   **TOTAL TIME:** 40 minutes

Gluten-free, Vegetarian

½ cup red quinoa

1 cup water

2 medium (about 2½-pound) acorn squash

1 tablespoon olive oil

1 clove garlic, minced

zest and juice of 1 lemon

¼ teaspoon salt

¼ teaspoon pepper

2 cups chopped kale

½ cup dried cranberries

¼ cup Parmesan cheese or dairy-free cheese

1. In a medium pot, add the quinoa and water, and bring to a boil. Reduce heat and simmer until quinoa is cooked through, about 15 minutes. Fluff the quinoa with a fork.

2. Using a knife, pierce the skin on both squash several times. Microwave for 18 minutes, rotating each halfway through. Carefully remove the squash and place them on a cutting board. Halve the squash lengthwise and use a spoon to scoop out the seeds.

3. In a medium bowl, whisk the oil, garlic, lemon zest and juice, salt, and pepper. Add the kale, tossing to combine.

4. Add the cooked quinoa and cranberries to the kale bowl, and stir to combine.

5. Scoop ½ cup of the quinoa mixture into each of the 4 squash halves, top with cheese, and serve.

Black Bean Quinoa Burgers

LUTEAL/PMS

Transforming iron-rich, plant-based proteins (like beans and quinoa) into a burger is an easy, delicious, and healthy way to support your cycle. The beans and quinoa sprinkle the body with energizing B vitamins, iron, zinc, and folate, all of which are instrumental for a healthy period and hormonal balance. This burger is great to help your body gear up for the upcoming phases so it may be in your best interest to double the recipe and freeze the extras for a nutritious, and quick dinner for the future!

SERVING SIZE: 4   **TOTAL TIME:** 30 minutes

Gluten-free, Dairy-free, Vegetarian

¼ cup quinoa

½ cup water

1 (15-ounce) can low-sodium black beans, drained and rinsed

1 medium carrot, grated

¼ cup old-fashioned oats

1 egg, beaten

¼ teaspoon salt

⅛ teaspoon pepper

1 tablespoon olive oil

1. In a medium saucepan over high heat, bring the quinoa and water to a boil. Reduce heat to low, cover, and simmer for 12 to 15 minutes, until all liquid has been absorbed. Remove from heat, and fluff the quinoa with a fork.

2. Place the black beans in a large bowl and mash with the back of a fork. Add the cooked quinoa, carrot, oats, egg, salt, and pepper, stirring to incorporate.

3. Scoop out ¼ cup of the quinoa mixture, and use clean hands to form it into a patty. Gently press down with the palm of your hand to form a disc, and place on a large plate. Repeat 3 more times with the remaining quinoa mixture.

4. In a large skillet over medium heat, heat the oil. When the oil is shimmering, place the patties into the oil, leaving ½ inch between each patty. Cook for about 8 minutes, flipping once, until the burgers are browned and cooked through.

5. Serve warm and drizzle preferred dressing/sauce on top.

Tip: Place cooled quinoa burgers in a freezer-safe container in the freezer for up to 2 months. To defrost, refrigerate overnight. Reheat one burger at a time in the microwave on high for 1 to 2 minutes. Burgers can also be reheated in a nonstick skillet over medium heat for about 5 minutes, flipping once.

Loaded Baked Sweet Potato with Beans

LUTEAL/PMS

SERVING SIZE: 2   **TOTAL TIME:** 90 minutes

Gluten-free, Vegetarian

POTATOES

2 medium sweet potatoes

1 tablespoon olive oil

2 cloves garlic, minced

2 cups diced cherry tomatoes

1 cup black beans

1 tablespoon apple cider vinegar

1 teaspoon brown miso paste

pinch of Himalayan salt

pinch of pepper

¼ teaspoon ground coriander

SOUR CREAM

1 cup 2 or 4% plain Greek yogurt or almond yogurt if dairy-free

1 tablespoon tahini

1 lemon, juiced

salt and pepper

GUACAMOLE

2 avocados, peeled and pitted

¼ teaspoon finely chopped fresh cilantro

½ lime, juiced

1 teaspoon garlic powder

¼ teaspoon paprika

½ teaspoon salt

1. Preheat the oven to 400°F.

2. Pierce the skin of the sweet potatoes and bake for an hour until cooked through.

3. Add the olive oil to a skillet over medium heat. After 2 minutes, add garlic and tomatoes, and mix together for 3 minutes, until garlic becomes fragrant.

4. Add the beans, apple cider vinegar, miso paste, salt, and pepper, and cook for 10 minutes on low-medium heat. Add the coriander toward the end.

5. Make the sour cream by mixing all the ingredients in a bowl until well combined.

6. Make the guacamole by mashing both avocados in a separate bowl. Mix in the cilantro, lime, garlic powder, paprika, and salt.

7. Remove the cooked sweet potatoes and cut in half. Remove most of the fleshy middle and mix with the beans and tomatoes.

8. Return the sweet potato, beans, and tomato mixture back into the crispy potato skin.

9. Top with the guacamole and sour cream.

Chicken and Strawberry Fields for Dinner

SERVING SIZE: 4   **TOTAL TIME:** 45 minutes

Gluten-free, Dairy-free

3 tablespoons olive oil

1 tablespoon apple cider vinegar

2 tablespoons lemon juice

1 tablespoon lime juice

¾ teaspoon kosher salt, divided

1 cup quartered strawberries

4 (4-ounce) boneless, skinless chicken breast or thigh

1 teaspoon chili powder

⅛ teaspoon crushed red pepper flakes

1 teaspoon coconut oil or olive oil

1 head bibb or gem lettuce, torn into large pieces

3 cups baby kale

¼ cup chopped cashews

1. Combine the olive oil, apple cider vinegar, lemon juice, lime juice and ¼ teaspoon of salt in a medium bowl. Add the strawberries, and stir to combine. Let sit for 15 minutes, stirring occasionally.

2. Meanwhile, sprinkle the chicken with the chili powder, crushed red pepper flakes, and the remaining ½ teaspoon of salt. Heat the coconut oil in a large skillet over medium-high for about 3 minutes.

3. Add the chicken to the skillet. Cook for 5 minutes per side, until the chicken is cooked through and no longer pink. Let stand for 5 minutes, then chop into small pieces.

4. Place the lettuce and kale on a platter. Toss with the chicken and strawberry dressing mixture, and then finish off with a sprinkle of cashews. Serve!

Vegetarian Quinoa Bowl with Kale and Roasted Vegetables

PMS is a time when cramps are in town, bloat is real, and you may not be your usual, awesome self. This recipe consolidates all the nutritional remedies to help you get through PMS like a champ. Pumpkin seeds will help squash bloat while providing potassium, a mineral that helps restore fluid balance in the body so you won't feel like a balloon. Mushrooms are high in vitamin D, known to help relieve cramps. You'll also get a nice boost of energy coming from iron sources kale and quinoa. Basically, this bowl will give you life.

SERVING SIZE: 2   **TOTAL TIME:** 40 minutes

Gluten-free, Dairy-free, Vegetarian

1 head broccoli, chopped into florets

1 medium red onion, sliced

1½ tablespoons olive oil, divided

salt and pepper, to taste

2 cups cremini or white mushrooms, sliced

2 cups quinoa, precooked

2 cups kale, chopped

2 servings of Maple Sunflower Seed Butter Lemon Dressing (page 255)

¼ cup pumpkin seeds (optional)

chopped herbs of choice (optional)

1. Preheat the oven to 400°F.

2. In a medium bowl, toss the broccoli and red onion with 1 tablespoon of olive oil, salt, and pepper.

3. Arrange the broccoli and onion in a single layer on a baking sheet and roast in the oven for 15 minutes, tossing occasionally, until tender and browned in places.

4. While the vegetables are roasting, heat a sauté pan over medium heat. Add the rest of the olive oil and the sliced mushrooms. Toss to coat the mushrooms in oil but do not add salt

(salt will cause the mushrooms to release their moisture and inhibit caramelization). Cook for 5 to 7 minutes, stirring occasionally until mushrooms are browned. Remove from the heat and then add a sprinkle of salt.

5. Build your bowl starting with a base of cooked quinoa grains. Add the chopped kale, roasted veggies, and caramelized mushrooms. Drizzle with a spoonful of Maple Sunflower Seed Butter Lemon Dressing, and top with the pumpkin seeds and herbs (such as basil, parsley, and/or chives), if using.

Cauliflower Grits

SERVING SIZE: 2   **TOTAL TIME:** 45 minutes

Gluten-free, Vegetarian

1½ cups cauliflower florets

1 teaspoon coconut oil

⅓ tablespoon plus 1 teaspoon almond flour

2 teaspoons coconut flour

1 teaspoon butter or olive oil, if dairy-free

½ cup almond milk

¼ teaspoon salt

⅛ teaspoon onion powder

⅛ teaspoon garlic powder

⅛ teaspoon pepper

⅓ cup grated cheddar cheese or dairy-free cheese, divided

1. Preheat the oven to 375°F.

2. Bring a large pot of salted water to a boil then add the cauliflower. Leave cauliflower in the water for about 7 minutes until fork-tender.

3. Drain the cauliflower and spread onto an absorbent towel. Gently press out the moisture from cauliflower onto the paper towel as much as possible.

4. Melt the coconut oil in a large pan over medium-high heat. When melted, add the almond flour, coconut flour, and butter or olive oil to pan. Whisk until browned, about 1 minute.

5. Add the milk, salt, onion powder, garlic powder, and pepper and whisk until smooth.

6. Bring the contents to a boil and then reduce to medium heat. Stir occasionally until thickened, about 8 minutes.

7. Remove the milk mixture from the heat and whisk in about two-thirds of the cheese until smooth.

8. Spread one-third of the sauce on the bottom of an 8 x 8-inch pan. Place the cauliflower in the pan on top of the mixture and spoon the rest of the sauce over the top. Sprinkle with the remaining cheese.

9. Bake until golden brown and bubbly, 7 to 10 minutes. Broil for 2 to 3 minutes until golden.

10. Let cool and serve.

Salmon and Shredded Brussels Sprout Tacos

These healthy tacos are such an easy and delicious dinner, you'll definitely make it part of your weekly dinner rotation. This dish does a great job balancing hormones thanks to the crunchy and refreshing Brussels sprouts. The omega-3-fatty acids coming from salmon will balance moodiness and hunger cravings, and can ward off anxiety and stress, especially when PMS strikes. Pair these PMS-friendly tacos with homemade guacamole and brown rice chips for a delightful dinner.

SERVING SIZE: 2   **TOTAL TIME:** 25 minutes

Gluten-free, Dairy-free

2 tablespoons lime juice

2 (4-ounce) salmon fillets

¼ teaspoon lemon pepper

½ teaspoon salt, divided

½ teaspoon chili powder, divided

2 tablespoons olive oil

3 cups raw, shredded Brussels sprouts

½ teaspoon onion powder

¼ teaspoon ground cumin

pinch of red pepper flakes

pinch of ground turmeric

4 coconut flour or cassava flour tortillas

2 tablespoons chopped fresh cilantro, to serve

1. Preheat the oven to 300°F.

2. Squeeze the lime juice over the salmon, then season with lemon pepper, ¼ teaspoon salt, and ¼ teaspoon chili powder.

3. Add 1 tablespoon of olive oil to a small skillet over medium heat. Allow the pan to warm for 2 to 3 minutes.

4. Place the seasoned fillets in the skillet skin-side up and cook 3 to 4 minutes on each side, until the inside is opaque and the fillets flake easily with a fork.

5. While the salmon is cooking, add the remaining tablespoon of olive oil to a medium skillet, then add the shredded Brussels sprouts.

6. Season with the onion powder, remaining ¼ teaspoon chili powder, cumin, red pepper flakes, turmeric, and remaining salt.

7. Cook until tender, 5 to 7 minutes.

8. Take the salmon off the heat, and separate into large pieces with a fork.

9. Add the cooked Brussels sprouts to the two tortillas, then place the pieces of salmon on top and garnish with cilantro.

10. Fold the tortillas into tacos and enjoy!

Easy Slow Cooker Lentil Soup

MENSTRUAL, OVULATORY, LUTEAL/PMS

Especially during your period when your body just doesn't feel up to par, there's nothing more soothing than a warm bowl of soup. Not only will this soup replenish the iron that you lost during your period, but you'll start to heal your gut with soothing and easy-to-digest bone broth. Lentils are high in fiber, hormone-balancing phytonutrients, and zinc, which is needed for healthy egg development. In fact, this soup works for pretty much any of the phases due to the flood of nutrients that balance hormones, moods, and digestion.

SERVING SIZE: 10   **TOTAL TIME:** 6 to 8 hours

Gluten-free, Dairy-free

6 cloves garlic minced

2 stalks celery, chopped

2 large onions, chopped

3 large carrots, chopped

2 tablespoons olive oil

1 (16-ounce) bag lentils, washed and drained

9½ cups water

4 beef bouillon or vegetable cubes

5 to 6 fresh basil leaves, chopped

1 (6-ounce) can tomato paste

¼ teaspoon dry rosemary

kosher salt and pepper

1. In a medium sauté pan, cook the garlic, celery, onions, and carrots in the olive oil until tender, roughly 5 to 7 minutes. Season with salt and pepper to taste.

2. Add the vegetable mixture to a 6-quart slow cooker with the rest of the ingredients and mix through.

3. Turn the slow cooker on high for 5 hours, and then turn down to low until ready to serve; or you can turn the slow cooker on medium for 7 to 8 hours.

4. Serve with your favorite veggie side dish, crackers, or bread.

Green Goddess Dressing

MENSTRUAL, FOLLICULAR, OVULATORY

SERVING SIZE: 2 **TOTAL TIME:** 5 minutes

Gluten-free, Dairy-free, Vegetarian

½ cup 88 Acres Pumpkin Seed Butter

½ cup chopped flat-leaf parsley

½ cup chopped fresh spinach

1 clove garlic, smashed

¼ cup roughly chopped shallots

juice of 1 lemon

1 teaspoon apple cider vinegar

1 teaspoon salt

½ teaspoon pepper

½ cup warm water, to thin*

1. In a large mixing bowl or blender, stir together all ingredients except the water until fully combined.

2. Slowly add the water in small increments, stirring in between additions, until you reach a pourable consistency.

3. Drizzle on a grain bowl, fresh salads, or grilled vegetables, or transfer to a jar, cover, and refrigerate for up to 1 week.

* Use less water to make a veggie dip consistency.

Maple Sunflower Seed Butter Lemon Dressing

SERVING SIZE: 2   **TOTAL TIME:** 5 minutes

Gluten-free, Dairy-free, Vegetarian

3 cloves garlic, grated

2 tablespoons olive oil

¼ cup lemon juice (from about 2 small lemons)

grated zest of 1 lemon

1 teaspoon kosher salt

½ cup 88 Acres Maple Sunflower Seed Butter

⅔ cup water, to thin

1. In a small bowl, combine the grated garlic and olive oil. Stir to combine, and let the garlic infuse the olive oil for about 15 minutes. Strain out the garlic and discard.

2. In a medium bowl, whisk the garlic-infused olive oil, lemon juice, lemon zest, and salt until combined. Add the seed butter, and stir to combine. The mixture will be very thick.

3. Slowly add the water to the seed butter mixture and whisk until smooth, adding more water until you reach the desired consistency.

4. Drizzle over a grain bowl, fresh salads, or grilled vegetables, or transfer to a jar, cover, and refrigerate for up to 1 week.

Tahini Dressing

SERVING SIZE: 2 **TOTAL TIME:** 5 minutes

Gluten-free, Dairy-free, Vegetarian

¼ cup tahini

1 teaspoon kosher salt

½ teaspoon garlic powder

⅛ cup warm water

1. Whisk all of the ingredients except the water in a bowl.

2. Slowly add the warm water while whisking to incorporate. Add more water until you reach the desired texture.

3. Add more salt or garlic powder based on your preference.

4. Serve on a salad or a meal, or transfer to a jar, cover, and refrigerate for up to 1 week.

Easy Peasy Parsley Dressing

SERVING SIZE: 2 **TOTAL TIME:** 5 minutes

Gluten-free, Dairy-free, Vegetarian

2 cups flat-leaf parsley, stems removed

½ teaspoon kosher salt

3 tablespoons lemon juice

1 clove garlic, crushed

½ cup olive oil

½ tablespoon champagne vinegar

1. Blend all of the ingredients in a food processor until smooth.

2. Serve on a salad, or transfer to a jar, cover, and refrigerate for up to 1 week.

DESSERT

Pumpkin Spice Blondies

SERVING SIZE: 16 squares **TOTAL TIME:** 45 minutes

Gluten-free, Dairy-free, Vegetarian

½ cup 88 Acres Vanilla Spice Sunflower Seed Butter

½ cup canned pumpkin puree

½ cup maple syrup

1 egg

1 teaspoon vanilla extract

2 tablespoons sunflower seed oil

1 cup oat flour

½ teaspoon baking powder

¼ teaspoon kosher salt

½ cup mini dark chocolate chips or dairy-free chocolate chips

1. Preheat the oven to 350°F. Line an 8 x 8-inch pan with parchment paper and set aside.

2. In a large bowl, combine the seed butter, pumpkin, maple syrup, egg, vanilla, and sunflower seed oil. Use a whisk or a hand mixer to blend the ingredients until completely smooth.

3. In a small bow, mix the oat flour, baking powder, and salt together. Add the dry ingredients to the wet ingredients, and stir to combine. Add the chocolate chips, and mix to distribute evenly.

4. Pour the mixture into the prepared pan, using a spatula to smooth the top. Bake for 25 to 30 minutes, until a toothpick inserted in the middle comes out clean. Cool to room temperature before cutting into pieces.

Dark Chocolate and Cranberry Fudge Bars

MENSTRUAL, LUTEAL/PMS

SERVING SIZE: 16 bars   **TOTAL TIME:** 2½ hours

Gluten-free, Vegetarian

CRUST

12 pitted Medjool dates

1½ cups sunflower seeds

2 tablespoons unsweetened cacao powder

¼ teaspoon salt

FILLING

1½ cups 88 Acres Dark Chocolate Sunflower Seed Butter

SUGARED CRANBERRIES

1 cup coconut or brown sugar, divided

½ cup water

1½ cups fresh cranberries

1. Add the crust ingredients to a food processor and blend until a loose dough forms. The dough should stick together when pinched between two fingers. If it's too dry, add another date or two.

2. Line an 8 x 8-inch baking pan with parchment paper, letting the excess hang over two sides. Press the dough firmly into the bottom of the pan, using more parchment or a flat-bottomed cup to get an even layer.

3. Cover the crust with the Dark Chocolate Sunflower Seed Butter and spread into an even layer. Refrigerate for at least 1 hour or until the seed butter is firm.

4. While the crust and filling are chilling, make the sugared cranberries. Dissolve ½ cup sugar into ½ cup water in a medium saucepan over low heat.

5. Remove the syrup from the heat and fold in the cranberries until evenly coated. Use a slotted spoon to remove the cranberries from the syrup. Let the cranberries dry on a cooling rack or parchment-lined baking sheet.

6. When the cranberries are completely dry, add the rest of the sugar to a shallow bowl or dish. Working in batches, toss the cranberries in the sugar, shaking off the excess before arranging them evenly on top of the Dark Chocolate Sunflower Seed Butter filling. Press the cranberries lightly into the filling with parchment paper and refrigerate for another hour before serving.

Date and Peanut Butter Frozen Bites

MENSTRUAL, LUTEAL/PMS

If you don't know what these frozen bites are, you aren't alone. These date bites are a triple threat; they satisfy your chocolate craving, deliver magnesium to relieve cramps, and are the perfect combo of salty and sweet. Plus, magnesium can help lower cortisol (your stress hormone) and stabilize blood sugars. Make a bunch ahead of time so you can store extras in your freezer whenever the mood strikes for the yummy perfect bite, without any guilt (or stress) whatsoever!

SERVING SIZE: 2   **TOTAL TIME:** 10 minutes

Gluten-free, Vegetarian

3 tablespoons creamy peanut butter

1 tablespoon coconut oil

3 tablespoons dark chocolate (or dairy-free dark chocolate chips), divided

6 large pitted Medjool dates, halved and pressed open

1. Mix the peanut butter and coconut oil in a medium bowl. (Try microwaving the coconut oil if it is hard prior to mixing.)

2. Place 2 tablespoons of chocolate in a small microwave-safe bowl, and melt in the microwave in 15-second increments until smooth.

3. Fill each date with the nut butter and drizzle with the chocolate.

4. Chop the remaining 1 tablespoon of chocolate and sprinkle over the top.

5. Place in a plastic container and freeze for 2 hours or until ready to eat.

Dark Chocolate Peanut Butter Cups

SERVING SIZE: 6 pieces   **TOTAL TIME:** 40 minutes plus 3 hours to freeze

Gluten-free, Vegetarian

½ cup dark chocolate chips or dairy-free dark chocolate chips

2 tablespoons peanut butter

2 tablespoons coconut oil

¼ teaspoon Himalayan salt

1. Place the chocolate chips in a small microwave-safe bowl, and melt in the microwave in 15-second increments until smooth.

2. Line a muffin tin with double-layered paper cups and place a small amount of the chocolate, enough to coat the sides, in the bottom of each cup.

3. Use a spoon or toothpick to push the chocolate up the sides of the paper cups to create a base.

4. Place the muffin tin in the freezer until hardened, about 15 minutes.

5. While the chocolate bases are freezing, make the peanut butter filling by mixing the peanut butter, coconut oil, and salt in a medium bowl.

6. Remove the muffin tin from the freezer and add a spoonful of the filling to the chocolate-layered paper cup.

7. Top each cup with the remaining melted chocolate.

8. Let the cups set in the freezer for up to 3 hours, then enjoy!

No-Bake Chocolate Peanut Butter Squares

SERVING SIZE: 16   **TOTAL TIME:** 40 minutes, including refrigeration

Gluten-free, Vegetarian

5 pitted Medjool dates

⅓ cup maple syrup

1⅛ cups creamy peanut butter

2½ cups old fashioned oats

¾ cup dark chocolate chips, or dairy-free chocolate chips

1. Blend the pitted dates, maple syrup, peanut butter, and oats until well combined.

2. Line a rimmed baking sheet with parchment paper.

3. Press the peanut butter-oat batter into a smooth layer on the baking sheet.

4. Melt the chocolate chips in a double boiler or in the microwave in 15-second intervals until melted.

5. Spread the melted chocolate on top, and place in the refrigerator to set and cool, 25 to 30 minutes.

6. Remove from the refrigerator and cut into squares. Store in the refrigerator for up to 5 days or freezer for 4 to 6 months.

Clementines and Dark Chocolate Fudge Sauce

This is a winning dessert combo and will arm your body with a good nutritional defense system. The magnesium and antioxidants coming from both dark chocolate and clementines (or orange sections if you can't find clementines) will help your body feel more relaxed during the physiological stress of PMS and menstruation. Dark chocolate also contains the amino acid arginine, which helps dilate tiny blood vessels and increases blood flow to the uterus, ovaries, and genitals. The more blood flow, the less muscle pain and cramping. Bonus, the increased blood flow may even amplify your desire for sex. Ooh la la!

SERVING SIZE: 2   **TOTAL TIME:** 35 minutes

Gluten-free, Vegetarian

½ cup 88 Acres Dark Chocolate Sunflower Seed Butter

½ cup almond milk or milk of choice

¼ cup dark chocolate chips or dairy-free dark chocolate chips

1 tablespoon butter, cut into small cubes

1 teaspoon vanilla extract

4 peeled clementines

½ teaspoon salt

1. Place the seed butter, chocolate chips, vanilla extract, and salt in a heat-proof bowl and set aside.

2. In a small saucepan, heat the milk on low until simmering, watching it closely so it does not reach a full boil.

3. Slowly pour the hot milk into the bowl with the chocolate chips, whisking constantly until the milk is fully incorporated and the sauce is smooth.

4. Add the butter, a few cubes at a time, whisking continuously until it is fully melted and combined.

5. Place the clementines on a parchment paper-lined baking sheet. Drizzle the sauce over the clementines. Serve warm or place in the refrigerator for 20 minutes to allow the sauce to harden.

RESOURCES

88 ACRES
https://88acres.com
This company's healthy snacks are natural, wholesome, gluten-free, nut-free, and non-GMO. They make craft seed bars, grainless seed'nola, and seed butters free of the top eight allergens.

AMERICAN THYROID ASSOCIATION (ATA)
www.thyroid.org
The ATA is dedicated to the advancement, understanding, prevention, diagnosis, and treatment of thyroid disorders and thyroid cancer.

AVA
https://www.avawomen.com
Ava is a wearable ovulation tracker that you wear on your wrist while you sleep for effortless insight about your fertility, pregnancy, and health. It monitors your skin temperature, resting pulse rate, breathing rate, heart rate variability ratio, and sleep.

AZO
https://www.azoproducts.com
AZO is an over-the-counter medication that provides fast relief from urinary pain, burning, urgency, and frequency associated with urinary tract infections. The company has a full line of products designed to help maintain urinary, vaginal, and bladder health.

BANZA
www.banza.com
Banza chickpea pasta is a high-protein, lower-carb, gluten-free alternative to traditional pasta. It is also allergen-free, high in fiber and protein, and free of added sugar in any of its products.

BLUME

https://www.meetblume.com

This e-commerce startup focuses on providing safe, sustainable period products for women and girls who believe in the power of their choices.

BONAFIDE

https://hellobonafide.com/products/serenol

Bonafide is a company that provides non-prescription solutions that treat women's health using ingredients from nature as often as possible to maximize effectiveness and relief.

CORA

https://cora.life

Cora is a menstrual product company that combines healthy, organic tampons, with modern design, an easy delivery system, and a globally conscious practice, all in one go. The tampons are 100% organic, biodegradable, hypoallergenic, BPA-free, and contain no fragrances or synthetics. With every Cora purchase, Cora provides pads and health education to a girl in need.

DAYSY

https://usa.daysy.me

Daysy is an intelligent fertility tracker that lets you get to know your very own menstrual cycle. Thanks to Daysy, you'll know exactly when you are in your fertile window and when you are not. Daysy fertility tracker is an easy way to track your menstrual cycle and identify your fertile phase.

ENDOMETRIOSIS FOUNDATION OF AMERICA

www.endofound.org

The Endometriosis Foundation of America strives to increase disease recognition, provide advocacy, facilitate expert surgical training, and fund landmark endometriosis research.

FOOD PERIOD

https://www.foodperiod.com

Food Period designs functional food products that support women's menstrual cycles naturally. Food Period is a subscription-based service that helps women use natural food products to improve their periods. Food Period's mission is to make natural solutions for hormonal health challenges more easily accessible to women.

KINDBODY

https://kindbody.com

Kindbody provides women's health and fertility services for the women of today. Kindbody offers a full suite of fertility and wellness services to support women at every step in their fertility journey.

NATIONAL ALLIANCE ON MENTAL ILLNESS (NAMI)

www.nami.org

The National Alliance on Mental Illness is a nationwide grassroots advocacy group representing people affected by mental illness in the United States. NAMI educates, supports, and advocates for people living with mental illnesses and their families.

NATIONAL EATING DISORDERS ASSOCIATION (NEDA)

www.nationaleatingdisorders.org

The National Eating Disorders Association is an American non-profit organization devoted to preventing eating disorders, providing treatment referrals, and increasing the education and understanding of eating disorders, weight, and body image.

PERIOD. END OF SENTENCE.
Netflix

An Oscar-winning Netflix original documentary short about a group of women who rise up against the stigma of menstruation, make low-cost sanitary pads on a new machine, and stride toward financial independence.

PERIOD MOVEMENT
www.period.org

Global, youth-powered nonprofit that strives to provide for menstruators in need through service, education, and policy.

PERIOD SPACE
http://periodspace.org

This online reproductive health resource and platform is aimed at destigmatizing periods and encouraging ongoing public discussion on menstruation. Period space is a safe space for people of all walks of life to learn more about their bodies and share their experiences, as well as open the conversation around periods and bleeding.

RAEL
https://www.getrael.com

Rael's mission is to provide natural and organic feminine care products that don't sacrifice comfort or functionality. Rael is centered around quality, performance, and convenience. Their vision is to empower and inform women with safer, healthier alternatives for their bodies.

RESOLVE: THE NATIONAL INFERTILITY ASSOCIATION
https://resolve.org

The National Infertility Association is a nationwide nonprofit dedicated to ensuring that all people challenged in their family-building journey reach resolution. RESOLVE provides free support groups in more than 200 communities; is the leading patient advocacy voice; and serves as the go-to organization for anyone challenged in their family building.

ROBYN
wearerobyn.co

Robyn is a partner in your unique journey to parenthood, providing access to integrative maternal wellness tools, resources, and providers while offering a community of support where you can share, learn, and grow.

THINX
https://www.shethinx.com

This company provides period-proof underwear that is washable and reusable. These undies absorb your period and are a more sustainable solution than single-use disposable products. Depending on your flow (light, medium, heavy), THINX can replace pads, tampons, liners, and cups, or can be worn with tampons and cups for extra protection.

TULA
https://www.tula.com

TULA is a skin company that uses probiotic technology. Their products are clean, cruelty-free, toxic-free, and combined with 100% natural probiotics with superfoods like blueberries, turmeric, and vitamin C. They also offer probiotic dietary supplements.

BOOKS

The Complete A to Z for Your V, by Dr. Alyssa Dweck and Robin Westen

Period Power, a Manifesto for the Menstrual Movement, by Nadya Okamoto

Run Fast. Cook Fast. Eat Slow., by Shalane Flanagan and Elyse Kopecky

INDEX

RECIPE INDEX

ACKNOWLEDGMENTS

This book would not have been possible without my team supporting me and, most importantly, cheering me on. A special thanks to my incredible research assistants and interns Niki Cohen, Jamie Gershel, and Mary Matone for putting hard work and dedication into each and every task thrown their way. A heartwarming thank you to Sarah Rueven, Leyla Bilali, and Dara Godfrey for lending me their expertise, support, and kindness always.

I'm so appreciative of Alyssa and Maria Tosoni of the incredible blog, Spinach4Breakfast, and rockstar food companies Banza and 88 Acres for their recipe contributions. You've opened my eyes (and my belly) to being creative and nutritious in the kitchen.

A big thank you to Allison Kasirer, founder of Robyn, for inspiring and teaching me that honesty and vulnerability pave the way for positive change and progression. A huge thank you to Dr. Alyssa Dweck for lending me her keen medical expertise in helping to shape this book into what it is today, and to my nutrition advisor and friend, Dr. Julie Thurlow, for always believing in me, even as a young student at the University of Wisconsin-Madison.

I'm eternally grateful for Kristen Mancinelli for making my dream of writing a book become a reality. Thank you to Sami Fishbein and Aleen Kuperman for looping me into the Betches empire and for steering me in the right direction with your savvy advice and guidance. I'm so grateful for your friendship, support, and ongoing kindness.

I couldn't have done this without Rachel Greenwald, my mentor and voice of reason. Big Rachel, you've taught me so many invaluable lessons about business, perseverance, and hard work. Everyone should have a Rachel Greenwald in their life, and I'm so fortunate that I actually do.

Thank you to my GalPals for motivating and cheering me on, you are all the best.

A tremendous thank you to Katelyn Dougherty, Alyssa Reuben, and Hannah Tenenbaum at Paradigm Talent Agency for your constant support, wisdom, and keen insight. You've helped to make this all possible and I know it's just the beginning.

Thanks to the incredible crew at Ulysses Press; your dedication and guidance are truly appreciated.

Mom and Dad, thank you for allowing me to be a picky eater as a kid (ew, no green things!) or else I may not have ended up in this "fruitful" career. You've always supported my passion toward nutrition and encouraged me to always do my best, no matter what. This book would not have happened without your wisdom, ongoing love, and impeccable editing skills.

Rachel and Sean, you've both been an invaluable sounding board, have given me so many pearls of wisdom, and I'm eternally grateful. Lily, thank you for listening, agreeing with all of my ideas, and being the perfect and cutest distraction.

Scott, your patience, flexibility, love, and never-ending support are the primary backbones that made this book possible. I can't thank you enough for letting me talk to you tirelessly about menstrual cycles and periods. You are the peanut butter to my jelly, I mean, the poached egg to my avocado toast! I love you lots.

ABOUT THE AUTHOR

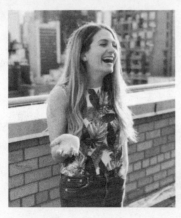

Tracy Lockwood Beckerman, MS, RD, CDN, is a leading women's health expert and nationally recognized registered dietitian. She received her bachelor's degree in nutritional sciences from the University of Wisconsin-Madison and her master's degree in clinical nutrition from New York University.

Her straightforward yet friendly and relatable voice has allowed her to break through the wellness space as a refreshing and honest nutrition expert. She influences millions through media with magazine and online features, podcasts, speaking engagements, and YouTube videos.

Tracy is the nutrition expert for Betches Media and appears regularly on their hit wellness podcast *Diet Starts Tomorrow*. Tracy is the host of *You Versus Food*, a food and nutrition YouTube series created by Well+Good, a health and wellness media company. Tracy also sits on the advisory board of Robyn, a company whose mission is to provide guidance and support across all paths to parenthood. She continues to grow her nutrition company, Tracy Nutrition, as well as her social media platform on Instagram as @thehappiestnutritionist.